Voice and Communication in Transgender and Gender Diverse Individuals

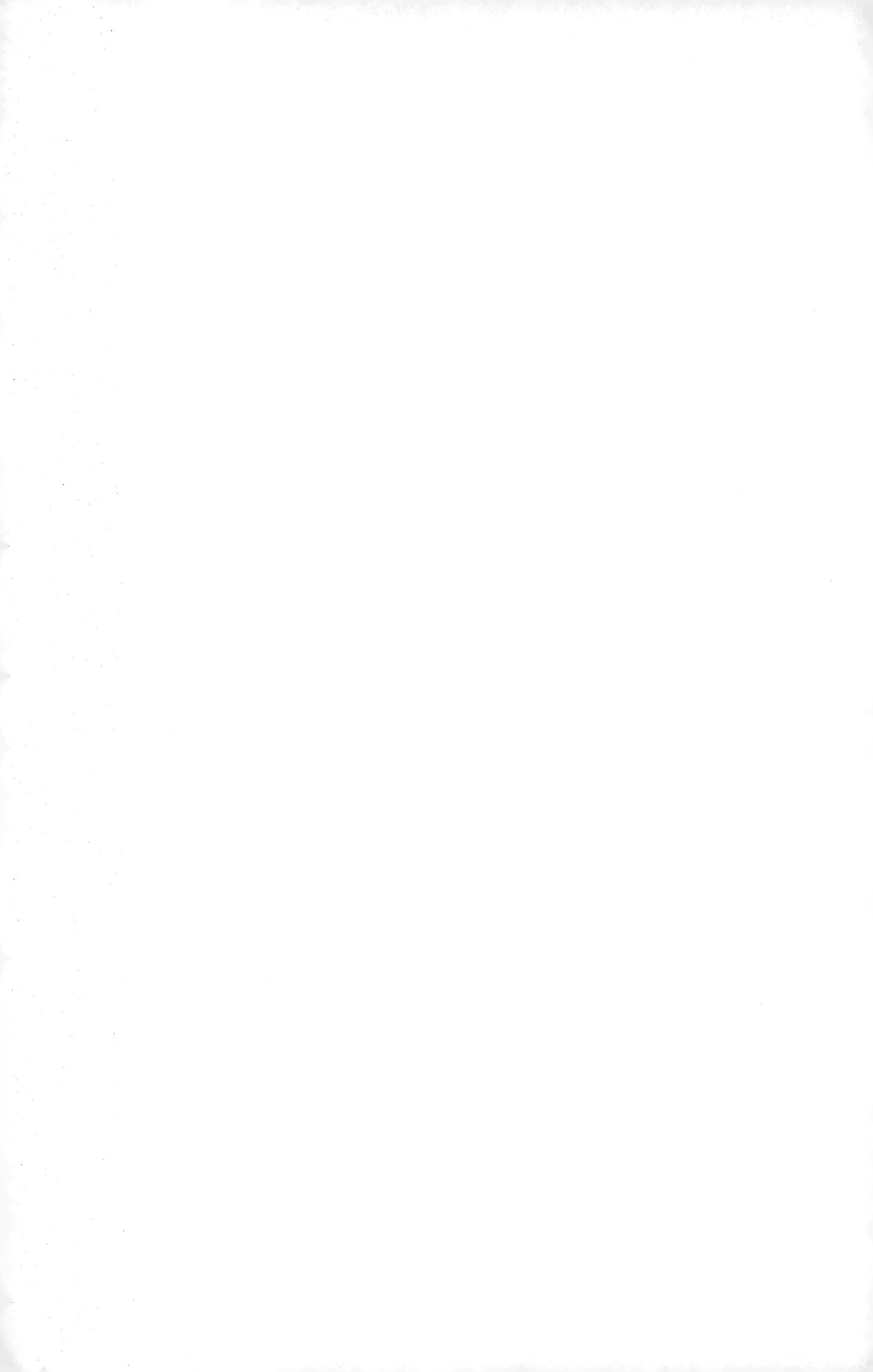

Mark S. Courey • Sarah K. Rapoport
Leanne Goldberg • Sarah K. Brown
Editors

Voice and Communication in Transgender and Gender Diverse Individuals

Evaluation and Techniques for Clinical Intervention

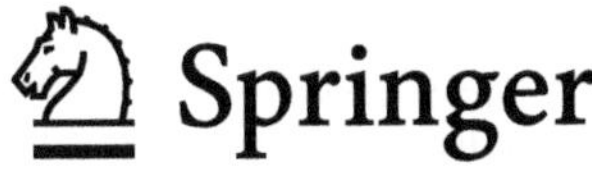

Editors
Mark S. Courey
Department of Otolaryngology/ Head and Neck Surgery
Mount Sinai Health System
New York, NY, USA

Sarah K. Rapoport
Department of Otolaryngology/Head and Neck Surgery
Georgetown University Hospital
Washington, D.C., DC, USA

Leanne Goldberg
Department of Otolaryngology/Head and Neck Surgery
Mount Sinai Health System
New York, NY, USA

Sarah K. Brown
SKB Voice Studio
New York, NY, USA

ISBN 978-3-031-24634-0 ISBN 978-3-031-24632-6 (eBook)
https://doi.org/10.1007/978-3-031-24632-6

This Springer imprint is published by the registered company Springer Nature Switzerland AG
The registered company address is: Gewerbestrasse 11, 6330 Cham, Switzerland

Preface

Thank you for your interest in our book entitled "The Management of Voice and Communication in Transgender and Gender Nonconforming Individuals: A Guide to Behavioral, Medical, and Surgical Therapies." Achieving a voice that is congruent with one's identity is an intricate and nuanced process for patients as well as the providers caring for them. The goal of this text is to bring together the leading clinicians who care for transgender and gender nonconforming individuals from behavioral, medical, and surgical perspectives and to impart the clinical expertise and experience they have developed surrounding voice care for this population. We have designed this book as a resource for otolaryngologists and speech-language pathologists as well as primary care providers, endocrinologists, and psychologists. We have attempted to synthesize the behavioral, clinical, and surgical management of transgender and gender nonconforming patients seeking voice change. We would like to thank the outstanding contributors to this work, which we believe fills a unique gap in otolaryngology. We hope that you, our reader, will find this work to be a valuable resource in your clinical practice.

New York, NY, USA — Mark S. Courey
Washington, DC, USA — Sarah K. Rapoport
New York, NY, USA — Leanne Goldberg
New York, NY, USA — Sarah K. Brown

Disclaimer

An all-inclusive list of gender terminology cannot exist given the constantly evolving definitions, titles, labels, and terms within the transgender and gender nonconforming (TGNC) community. Any list of TGNC-related terms must therefore be routinely updated. The terms used in this text were current at the time the book was written and are meant to be inclusive in the patients they reference.

Contents

Part I Background: Patient History and Evaluation

1 **Introduction to the Care of Transgender Persons** 3
Joshua D. Safer

2 **Medical Management for Transgender Patients** 7
Tamar Reisman and Roy Zucker

3 **Strategies for Evaluating Patients' Readiness for Surgical Intervention: From a Psychiatric Perspective** 17
Max Lichtenstein

4 **Barriers to Care and Cultural Responsiveness in Transgender and Gender Nonconforming Voice Modification** 27
A. C. Goldberg and Ruchi Kapila

5 **Patient-Reported Outcomes and Data Collection in Treatment-Seeking Transgender and Gender Nonconforming Individuals** 43
Maurice E. Goodwin, Ruchi Kapila, and Ry Pilchman

Part II Behavioral Interventions to Aid Transition

6 **Applying Flow Phonation in Voice Care for Transgender Women, Nonbinary, and Gender Nonconforming Individuals** 65
Sarah L. Schneider

7 **Resonant Voice Care** 79
Tina Babajanians

8 **Working with Pitch in Transgender and Gender Nonconforming Voice Care** 89
Christella Antoni

9 **Nonverbal Communication** 103
Ali Heitzman, Libby Lavella Perfitt, and Aaron Ziegler

10 **The Singing Voice** 113
Felix A. Graham

11 **Behavioral Management for Masculinization of Voice and Communication Across the Gender Spectrum** 135
Olivia Boddicker and Rachel Kominsky

Part III Surgical Techniques to Aid Transition

12 **Surgical Concepts in Transgender Voice Change** 157
Sarah K. Rapoport and Sarah K. Brown

13 **Cricothyroid Approximation** 161
Chadwan Al Yaghchi, Christella Antoni, and Guri Sandhu

14 **Laser-Assisted Voice Adjustment (LAVA)** 169
Brian Nuyen and Lisa A. Orloff

15 **Laser Reduction Glottoplasty: Vocal Fold Reduction Surgery for Feminine Voice Quality in Transgender Women** 177
İsmail Koçak and Okan Övünç

16 **Modified Wendler Glottoplasty: Endoscopic Bilateral Partial Cordectomy with Primary Closure** 187
Sarah K. Rapoport and Mark S. Courey

17 **Feminization Laryngoplasty** 197
James P. Thomas

18 **Type III Thyroplasty: Voice Masculinization** 207
Vyas Prasad and Marc Remacle

19 **Thyroid Cartilage Reduction** 217
Joseph Chang

Index 225

Contributors

Chadwan Al Yaghchi Imperial College Healthcare NHS Trust, London, UK

Christella Antoni Voice and Speech Services, University College London (UCL), London, UK

University College London, London, UK

Tina Babajanians Newport Beach, CA, USA

Olivia Boddicker Department of Otolaryngology, Grabscheid Voice and Swallowing Center of Mount Sinai, New York, NY, USA

Sarah K. Brown Speech Pathologist and Singing Voice Specialist, SKB Voice Studio, New York, NY, USA

Joseph Chang Department of Otolaryngology- Head and Neck Surgery, University of Washington, Seattle, WA, USA

Mark S. Courey Department of Otolaryngology Head and Neck Surgery, Division of Laryngology, Mount Sinai Health System, New York, NY, USA

A. C. Goldberg Transplaining LLC, Massachusetts Public Schools, The CREDITs Institute, Cambridge, MA, USA

Maurice E. Goodwin Houston Methodist's Department of Otolaryngology—Head and Neck Surgery, Houston Methodist Hospital, Houston, TX, USA

Felix A. Graham Independent Scholar, New York, NY, USA

Ali Heitzman Outpatient, UCLA, Los Angeles, CA, USA

Ruchi Kapila Kapila Voice and Speech Services, Hayward, CA, USA

İsmail Koçak DrVoice Clinic (Private Practise), Istanbul, Turkey

Rachel Kominsky, MD Division of Laryngology, Department of Otorhinolaryngology—Head and Neck Surgery, Montefiore Medical Center, Bronx, NY, USA

Libby Lavella Perfitt Singuistics, Pinole, CA, USA

Max Lichtenstein Department of Psychiatry, Icahn School of Medicine, New York, NY, USA

Brian Nuyen Department of Otolaryngology-Head and Neck Surgery, Stanford University School of Medicine, Stanford, CA, USA

Department of Otolaryngology-Head and Neck Surgery, Stanford University School of Medicine, Stanford, CA, USA

Lisa A. Orloff Division of Head and Neck Surgery, Department of Otolaryngology-Head and Neck Surgery, Stanford University School of Medicine, Stanford, CA, USA

Okan Övünç Tekirdag State Hospital Otorhinolaryngology Department, Tekirdag, Turkey

Ry Pilchman Rutgers University, Newark, NJ, USA

Robert Wood Johnson Barnabas Health, New Brunswick, NJ, USA

Prismatic Speech Services, New York, NY, USA

Vyas Prasad Singapore Medical Specialist Centre, Otolaryngology-Head and Neck Surgery, Singapore, Singapore

Sarah K. Rapoport Department of Otolaryngology/Head & Neck Surgery, Washington DC Veterans Affairs Medical Center; Georgetown University Hospital, Washington, DC, USA

Tamar Reisman Mount Sinai Hospital, New York, NY, USA

Marc Remacle Department of ORL-Head & Neck Surgery, Centre Hospitalier Luxembourg—Eich, Luxembourg, Luxembourg

Joshua D. Safer Mount Sinai Center for Transgender Medicine and Surgery, Mount Sinai Health System, New York, NY, USA

Guri Sandhu Imperial College Healthcare NHS Trust, London, UK

Sarah L. Schneider Department of Otolaryngology Head and Neck Surgery, University of California San Francisco, San Francisco, CA, USA

James P. Thomas Laryngology, Voicedoctor Private Practice, Portland, OR, USA

Aaron Ziegler Wellness Group for Voice, Speech, and Swallowing, LLC, Portland, OR, USA

Roy Zucker LGBT+ Health services, Tel Aviv Sourasky Medical Center, Tel Aviv-Yafo, Israel

Part I
Background: Patient History and Evaluation

Chapter 1
Introduction to the Care of Transgender Persons

Joshua D. Safer

Gender identity is the term for people's internal sense of their own sex: male, female, neither, or a combination of both (Table 1.1). Transgender and gender non-binary people have gender identities that differ from their sex recorded at birth. Sex recorded at birth is usually determined when external genitalia are visualized. The most current reported data demonstrate that approximately 0.6% of the adult population, or 1.4 million persons, in the United States are TGNB [1].

Gender expression is the term for how people signal gender identity to themselves or to others. And gender expression is often signaled through appearance, clothing, or actions of various sorts.

There are multiple adjectives for people with gender identities that differ from their sex recorded at birth, including the following: trans, transgender, transsexual, gender non-binary, gender incongruent, and genderqueer. In current use, trans, transgender, and the acronym TGNB (transgender and non-binary) are all used as umbrella terms for all people for whom external genitalia at birth and gender identity are not aligned.

Cis or cisgender are adjectives for people who are not TGNB. Thus, cisgender people are those whose gender identities align with their sex recorded at birth.

People with male gender identity who were noted at birth to be female are often called trans men, transgender men, or transmasculine people. People with female gender identity who were noted at birth to be male are often called trans women, transgender women, or transfeminine people.

Gender dysphoria is a mental health diagnosis listed in the current International Classification of Diseases—version 10 (ICD-10) used to describe the discomfort felt by some TGNB people due to the lack of alignment between their visible anatomy and their gender identity. However, many TGNB people who seek medical

J. D. Safer (✉)
Mount Sinai Center for Transgender Medicine and Surgery, Mount Sinai Health System, New York, NY, USA

M. S. Courey et al. (eds.), *Voice and Communication in Transgender and Gender Diverse Individuals*, https://doi.org/10.1007/978-3-031-24632-6_1

Table 1.1 Definitions. (Adapted from Ref. [1])

Terms	Definitions
Sex/gender	Umbrella terms both for biologic characteristics and for stereotypical behaviors considered male, female, both, or neither
Gender identity	An individual's internal sense of one's own sex
Gender expression	How a person communicates gender identity internally and to others
Sexual orientation	An individual's internal romantic or sexual attraction to other people
Transgender, transsexual, trans, gender non-binary, gender incongruent, genderqueer	A list of adjectives for people whose gender identity differs from sex recorded at birth
Cisgender, non-transgender	Terms to reference people with gender identity aligned with sex recorded at birth
Gender-affirming or gender-confirming hormone treatment and surgery	Medical/surgical interventions designed to align the body with the gender identity
Gender dysphoria	A mental health term for the discomfort felt by some transgender people
Gender role	The expectations a society places on someone of a given gender. Transgender people often face rejection or discrimination when they do not conform to the gender role they are assigned at birth
Sex assigned/registered at birth, sometimes abbreviated to sex	A person's sex, male or female, registered at the time of birth usually based off of assessment of a newborn's primary sex characteristics. "Biological sex" is sometimes used but is not preferred as it incorrectly links "biology" to a male or female exclusive binary

interventions to align their bodies with their gender identities do not suffer from dysphoria. Still, many payers throughout the world insist on a gender dysphoria label in order to permit cost coverage for gender-affirming medical care [2]. When the ICD-11 is published, it will include a new diagnostic code for TGNB people labeled "gender incongruence." The new label will appear in a new diagnosis section addressing sexual health [3].

The current model for reproductive physiology among humans includes a significant biological component underlying gender identity [4]. Data supporting the biological underpinning to gender identity can be separated into several broad categories in order of the strength of evidence in each category:

1. Attempts to manipulate gender identity among intersex people (also labeled people with DSD for differences of sexual development) by external means have not been successful [5, 6].
2. When TGNB people have twins, a twin is more likely to also be transgender if they are identical twins than if they are fraternal twins [7].
3. More male gender identity is observed among XX chromosome individuals with virilizing congenital adrenal hyperplasia and exposure to excess androgen in

utero than is observed among the general population of people with XX chromosomes [8].

4. Individuals with complete androgen insensitivity syndrome (who have XY chromosomes) have female gender identity [9].

The majority of TGNB individuals present to clinicians in late adolescence or adulthood. However, despite the late presentation, many TGNB individuals report that their awareness of their gender incongruence began much earlier in life.

Other than a suggestion that there may be some influence from androgens on gender identity for at least some people, the data for biological underpinnings to gender identity shed little light on the mechanisms by which such biology would exert its influence. However, along with greater social awareness, the acceptance of the biological model has provided a basis for the focus on treatment to align the bodies of transgender people with their gender identities.

Many transgender persons experience barriers to healthcare access and medical mistreatment. As many as one in four TGNB patients reports, they have been denied medical services, while one in three TGNB patients reports avoiding care due to fear of discrimination [10, 11]. These barriers to care are thought to play a substantial role in the health disparities between transgender and cisgender persons, with higher rates of substance abuse, infection, mental health conditions, and cancer in transgender persons [11]. Improvement in access to medical care will require the participation of more general providers outside specialized settings. A central purpose of this text is to educate providers of TGNB patients seeking voice change with how to best provide successful voice care in an effort to optimize treatment while limiting such prejudices.

References

1. Safer JD, Tangpricha V. Care of the transgender patient. Ann Intern Med. 2019;171(1):ITC1–16.
2. Accessing Coverage for Transition-Related Health Care [Internet]. Lambda Legal 2020 [cited 2020 Jul 7]. https://www.lambdalegal.org/know-your-rights/article/trans-health-care
3. ICD-11: Classifying disease to map the way we live and die [Internet]. WHO | Regional Office for Africa. [cited 2021 Apr 29]. https://www.afro.who.int/news/icd-11-classifying-disease-map-way-we-live-and-die
4. Klein P, Narasimhan S, Safer JD. The Boston medical center experience: an achievable model for the delivery of transgender medical care at an academic medical center. Transgend Health. 2018;3(1):136–40.
5. Meyer-Bahlburg HFL. Gender identity outcome in female-raised 46,XY persons with penile agenesis, cloacal exstrophy of the bladder, or penile ablation. Arch Sex Behav 2005;34(4):423–438.
6. Reiner WG, Gearhart JP. Discordant sexual identity in some genetic males with cloacal exstrophy assigned to female sex at birth. N Engl J Med. 2004;350(4):333–41.
7. Heylens G, De Cuypere G, Zucker KJ, Schelfaut C, Elaut E, Vanden Bossche H, et al. Gender identity disorder in twins: a review of the case report literature. J Sex Med. 2012;9(3):751–7.

8. Dessens AB, Slijper FME, Drop SLS. Gender dysphoria and gender change in chromosomal females with congenital adrenal hyperplasia. Arch Sex Behav. 2005;34(4):389–97.
9. Mazur T. Gender dysphoria and gender change in androgen insensitivity or micropenis. Arch Sex Behav. 2005;34(4):411–21.
10. Reisner SL, Poteat T, Keatley J, et al. Global health burden and needs of transgender populations: a review. Lancet. 2016;388:412–36.
11. Jaffee KD, Shires DA, Stroumsa D. Discrimination and delayed health care among transgender women and men: implications for improving medical education and health care delivery. Med Care. 2016;54:1010–6.

Chapter 2
Medical Management for Transgender Patients

Tamar Reisman and Roy Zucker

Introduction

Although not all transgender patients seek medical intervention, for select individuals, hormone therapy is appropriate. Initial treatment for transgender adolescents includes puberty blockade, often followed by hormone therapy at age 16 that then continues throughout adulthood. Since such treatments may reduce a patient's fertility, consideration of fertility preservation should always be discussed prior to initiation of any hormonal or medical intervention. Age-appropriate malignancy screening should be also performed per current guidelines based on a patient's innate sexual organs regardless of hormone status.

Diagnosis and Decision to Begin Treatment

Hormone treatment can be both safe and effective in aligning a patient's body to their experienced gender. Additionally, medical and surgical interventions have been shown to improve transgender patients' quality of life [1, 2]. The *Diagnostic and Statistical Manual of Mental Disorders* (DSM-V) defines gender dysphoria as a transgender identity that is "associated with clinically significant distress or impairment in social, occupational, or other important areas of functioning" [3]. However, it is important to note that not every gender non-conforming individual

T. Reisman (✉)
Mount Sinai Hospital, New York, NY, USA
e-mail: tamar.reisman@mssm.edu

R. Zucker
LGBT+ Health services, Tel Aviv Sourasky Medical Center, Tel Aviv-Yafo, Israel
e-mail: RoyZ@tlvmc.gov.il

M. S. Courey et al. (eds.), *Voice and Communication in Transgender and Gender Diverse Individuals*, https://doi.org/10.1007/978-3-031-24632-6_2

experiences gender dysphoria. In the context of our evolving social culture, only *some* gender non-conforming individuals experience significant gender dysphoria at *some* point in their lifetimes [4].

Gender identity is durable, meaning that it does not change over time. There is no credible data demonstrating that it is possible to change a person's gender identity. Any attempts to change gender identity rely on pressure to conform to sexual norms [5] and risk resulting in poor psychosocial outcomes [6].

Before starting hormone therapy, a diagnosis of gender dysphoria should be made by the prescribing clinician. Gender incongruence is typically self-reported by the patient and does not necessarily need to be confirmed by a mental health professional [7]. In the cases of extenuating circumstances, such as the presence of untreated psychosis, the diagnosis of gender incongruence can be made by a qualified medical provider based on guidelines set forth by the World Professional Association for Transgender Health (WPATH) or the Global Endocrine Society [3, 7, 8]. Assessments of a patient's readiness for hormone therapy should be contingent upon assessing the patient's ability to provide informed consent. Complicating medical and mental health disorders should be stabilized prior to treatment [7].

The Management of Children and Adolescents

The medical management of transgender children and adolescents utilizes a puberty-delaying approach using puberty blockers in a fashion similar to the medical approach to treating patients with precocious puberty. Evidence in the medical literature demonstrates that younger children who identify as transgender may not necessarily identify as transgender when they reach adolescence, whereas transgender adolescents are likely to have persistent gender identities and become transgender adults [9, 10]. Therefore, due to the challenges in making a reliable transgender diagnosis in children, more permanent treatments for pediatric patients are typically not initiated until later in adolescence. Puberty suppression via gonadotropin-releasing hormone (GnRH) analogs can be started at Tanner stages 2–3. Since puberty suppression is fully reversible, it grants the patient and practitioner team time to determine whether hormone therapy should subsequently be initiated. Puberty suppression increases patient quality of life and cognitive functioning while decreasing emotional and behavioral instability [11]. Permanent surgeries are usually deferred until patients are able to consent (e.g., at age 18) [12].

Fertility Preservation

Both medical and surgical transgender treatments are potentially destructive of fertility. Thus, it is imperative to discuss fertility preservation with patients prior to the initiation of therapy. Currently it is not possible for patients to undergo sperm banking or oocyte cryopreservation prior to the onset of puberty [9]. The decision to delay treatment and allow the patient to go through their endogenous puberty for fertility preservation must be weighed against the benefits of initiating hormone therapy, particularly if the patient's gender dysphoria is severe and the need for treatment is urgent.

Hormone Therapy for Transgender Individuals

The current general strategies for hormone therapy for transgender patients include (1) androgens to virilize transgender men and (2) estrogens and anti-androgens to reduce testosterone levels to the conventional female range for transgender women [1, 7].

Hormone Therapy for Transgender Women: Male to Female (MTF)

Hormone therapy for transgender women aims to decrease testosterone to the female range (<100 ng/dL) while avoiding supra-physiological levels of estradiol (>200 pg/mL). Treatment regimens typically combine an estrogen-based therapy with an anti-androgen therapy. The results that patients can anticipate from these medications include decreased facial/body hair, decreased libido, decreased spontaneous erections, decreased skin oiliness, decreased muscle mass, redistribution of fat, and breast development within the first 3–12 months. Breast growth typically peaks after 2 years of hormone therapy [13]. Non-binary, transfeminine individuals may choose to be treated with feminizing hormones at smaller doses than typically used with transgender women.

Treatment with estradiol in and of itself suppresses testosterone levels in transgender women. However, giving a concomitant anti-androgen allows for lower doses of estrogen to be used, thus limiting dose-related adverse effects (Tables 2.1,

Table 2.1 Monitoring for transgender women (MTF) on hormone therapy

1. Monitor for feminizing and adverse effects every 3 months for the first year and then every 6–12 months
2. Monitor serum testosterone and estradiol at follow-up visits with a practical target in the female range (testosterone <50 ng/dL; E2 < 200 pg/mL)
3. Monitor prolactin and triglycerides before starting hormones and at follow-up visits
4. Monitor potassium levels if the patient is taking spironolactone
5. Obtain BMD screening before starting hormones for patients at risk for osteoporosis. Otherwise, start screening at age 60 or earlier if sex hormone levels are consistently low
6. Screen MTF patients for breast and prostate cancer appropriately

Table adapted from: Gardner I, Safer J. Progress on the road to better medical care for transgender patients. *Curr Opin Endocrinol Diabetes Obes* 2013; 20(6):55308

Table 2.2 Hormone regimes for transgender women

1. Anti-androgen
• Spironolactone [trade names include CaroSpir and Aldactone]
100–200 mg/day (up to 400 mg)
• Cyproterone acetate [trade names include Androcur, Androcur depot, Cyprostat, and Siterone]
50–100 mg/day
• Gonadotropin-releasing hormone (GnRH) agonists [trade names include Lupron, Zoladex, Trelstar, Viadur, and Eligard]
3.75 mg subcutaneous monthly
2. Oral estrogen
• Oral conjugated estrogens [trade names include Premarin, Cenestin, and Enjuvia]
2.5–7.5 mg/day
• Oral 17-beta estradiol
2–6 mg/day
3. Parenteral estrogen
• Estradiol valerate [trade names include Delestrogen, Progynon depot, and Progynova]
5–20 mg i.m./2 weeks or cypionate *2–10 mg i.m./week*
4. Transdermal estrogen [trade names include Alora, Climara, Divigel, Elestrin, Esclim, Estraderm, Estrasorb, and EstroGel]
• Estradiol patch
0.1–0.4 mg/2X week

Table adapted from: Gardner I, Safer J. Progress on the road to better medical care for transgender patients. *Curr Opin Endocrinol Diabetes Obes* 2013; 20(6):55308

2.2, and 2.3). Spironolactone is an aldosterone receptor antagonist that has been shown to decrease mortality in patients with New York Heart Association class 3 and greater congestive heart failure [14]. Spironolactone also inhibits the secretion and activity of testosterone (although the mechanism is not known). Because of its low cost and high safety profile, it is a very commonly used anti-androgen in the United States.

Spironolactone can be administered in doses of 100–200 mg daily, with doses up to 400 mg administered if tolerated. Adverse effects are dose-dependent, and the weak diuretic properties of spironolactone may become more apparent at higher doses. Doses may be divided, keeping in mind that evening dosing may result in nocturia. GnRH agonists such as leuprolide (3.75 mg subcutaneously monthly or 11.25 mg subcutaneously every 3 months) inhibit the production of luteinizing hormone (LH), follicle-stimulating hormone (FSH), and testosterone but are often expensive and must be given by subcutaneous injection. Although GnRH agonists have been used to treat children with precocious puberty along with adolescent transgender individuals and appear to be well-tolerated, there are no studies demonstrating safety with very long-term use. Cyproterone acetate is often used in Europe but is not available in the United States.

Estrogen can be administered orally, transdermally, or parenterally (Tables 2.1, 2.2, and 2.3). Oral conjugated estrogens in doses of 2.5–7.5 mg and oral 17-beta

Table 2.3 Adverse effects: anti-androgen and estrogen supplementation

Likely increased risk
Venous thromboembolic disease
Gallstones
Weight gain
Hypertriglyceridemia
Likely increased risk with the presence of additional risk factors
Cardiovascular disease
Possible increased risk
Hypertension
Hyperprolactinemia
Possible increased risk with the presence of additional risk factors
Type 2 diabetes mellitus
No increased risk or inconclusive
Breast cancer

Table adapted from: World Professional Association for Transgender Health. Standards of care for the health of transsexual, transgender, and gender non-conforming people. 7th ed.; 2011

estradiol in doses of 2–6 mg daily are popular because they are easy to use and readily available. With conjugated estrogens some metabolites are undetectable on serum estradiol tests. Ethinyl estradiol is not recommended as it has been associated with an increased risk of venous thromboembolism [15]. Some propose that the hepatic first pass for oral estrogen increases thrombosis risk and that a transdermal estradiol patch dosed at 0.1–0.4 mg twice weekly should be used in transgender women who are at increased risk for thromboembolic disease. Estradiol can be administered parenterally with estradiol valerate or cypionate dosed at 5–20 mg IM every 2 weeks or 2–10 mg IM every week, but these medication levels are more difficult to monitor.

Transgender women on hormone therapy should be monitored for feminizing and adverse effects every 3 months for the first year and then every 6–12 months (Tables 2.4, 2.5, and 2.6). Serum testosterone and estradiol levels should be monitored until they stabilize within the female range (testosterone <100 ng/dL; estradiol <200 pg/mL). Spironolactone is a potassium-sparing diuretic and can cause hyperkalemia in rare individuals, so it is vital to monitor potassium for patients taking spironolactone. Estrogen-sensitive markers such as prolactin and triglycerides are often monitored. Patients should be warned of the risk of venous thromboembolism [16], as well as the need for sufficient levels of sex hormones to maintain bone mass. Patients should therefore avoid hypogonadism, particularly those who have undergone orchiectomy or vaginoplasty. Bone mineral density screening should be initiated at age 60 but may be performed earlier if sex hormone levels prove to be persistently low [12, 13].

Table 2.4 Monitoring for transgender men (FTM) on hormone therapy

1. Monitor for virilizing and adverse effects every 3 months for the first year and then every 6–12 months
2. Monitor serum testosterone at follow-up visits with a practical target in the male range (300–1000 ng/dl). Peak levels for patients taking parenteral testosterone can be measured 24–48 h after injection. Trough levels can be measured immediately before injection
3. Monitor hematocrit and lipid profile before starting hormones and at follow-up visits
4. Bone mineral density (BMD) screening before starting hormones for patients at risk for osteoporosis. Otherwise, screening can start at age 60 or earlier if sex hormone levels are consistently low
5. Screen FTM patients with cervixes or breasts (pap smear, mammography)

Table adapted from: Gardner I, Safer J. Progress on the road to better medical care for transgender patients. *Curr Opin Endocrinol Diabetes Obes* 2013; 20(6):55308.

Table 2.5 Hormone regimes for transgender men

1. Oral
• Testosterone undecanoate [trade names include Andriol, Androxon, Aveed, Cernos Depot, Jatenzo, Nebido, Nebido-R, Panteston, Reandron 1000, Restandol, Undecanoate 250, and Undestor]
160–240 mg/day
2. Parenteral (intramuscular or subcutaneous)
• Testosterone enanthate or cypionate [trade names include Veed, depo-testosterone, Delatestryl, and Testopel]
50–200 mg/week or *100–200 mg/2 weeks*
• Testosterone undecanoate [trade names include Andriol, Androxon, Aveed, Cernos Depot, Jatenzo, Nebido, Nebido-R, Panteston, Reandron 1000, Restandol, Undecanoate 250, and Undestor]
1000 mg/12 weeks
3. Transdermal
• Testosterone 1% gel *2.5–10 g/day*
• Testosterone patch *2.5–7.5 mg/day*

Table adapted from: Gardner I, Safer J. Progress on the road to better medical care for transgender patients. *Curr Opin Endocrinol Diabetes Obes* 2013; 20(6):55308

While it is suspected that estrogens may increase the incidence of venous thromboembolic disease, hypertriglyceridemia, cardiovascular disease, hypertension, and hyperprolactinemia, the degree of risk remains an area for future study [1].

Table 2.6 Adverse effects: androgen supplementation

Likely increased risk
Polycythemia
Weight gain
Acne
Androgenic alopecia (balding)
Sleep apnea
Possible increased risk
Hyperlipidemia
Possible increased risk with the presence of additional risk factors
Destabilization of psychiatric disorders with manic or psychotic symptoms (bipolar, schizoaffective disorder)
Cardiovascular disease
Hypertension
Type 2 diabetes mellitus
No increased risk or inconclusive
Loss of bone density
Breast cancer
Cervical cancer
Ovarian cancer
Uterine cancer

Table adapted from: World Professional Association for Transgender Health. Standards of care for the health of transsexual, transgender, and gender non-conforming people. 7th ed.; 2011

Perioperative Hormone Management

In the past it was recommended that transgender women stop taking hormones prior to gender-affirming surgery due to the link between estrogen and venous thromboembolism. However, recent data suggests that there is no need to stop hormones preoperatively [17]. Transfeminine patients should be instructed to discontinue their anti-androgens following vaginoplasty and/or orchiectomy.

Hormone Therapy for Transgender Men: Female to Male (FTM)

The hormonal treatment for transgender men is analogous to hormone replacement therapy for hypogonadal cisgender men [1, 7]. The dose of testosterone is titrated to achieve a mid-normal male physiological range (300–1000 ng/dL). Hormone therapy results in facial/body hair growth, male-pattern balding, increased acne, increased libido, increased muscle mass, clitoromegaly, deepening of the voice, and redistribution of fat within the first 3–12 months of testosterone therapy. Menstrual cessation occurs in the majority of individuals after 6 months of treatment [18].

Testosterone can be administered orally, transdermally, or parenterally (Tables 2.4, 2.5, and 2.6). Testosterone enanthate or cypionate dosed at 50–200 mg weekly can be administered intramuscularly or subcutaneously [19]. Higher doses (100–200 mg) can be administered every 2 weeks but may result in more significant fluctuations in testosterone levels. Transdermal preparations such as testosterone gel (dose ranges 2.5–10 g/day) or testosterone patch (dose ranges 2.5–7.5 mg/day) will achieve the same virilizing effects as intramuscular testosterone, but the patch may cause skin irritation. Oral testosterone undecanoate (dose ranges 160–240 mg/day) was approved for use in the United States in 2019 [15]. There is no indication for concomitant treatment with anti-estrogens. Patients who identify as non-binary may choose to be treated with smaller doses of testosterone, which can be determined on a case-by-case basis. Patients taking testosterone should be monitored for both virilizing and adverse effects every 3 months for the first year and then every 6–12 months thereafter (Tables 2.4, 2.5, and 2.6).

Serum testosterone levels should be followed to ensure that they remain within the normative goal range. Patients taking testosterone enanthate or cypionate intramuscularly or subcutaneously can have testosterone peak levels measured 24–48 h after injections and intermittent trough levels measured immediately prior to injections. Patients taking testosterone transdermally can have levels sampled any time beginning 1 week after administration. Androgen-sensitive indices such as hematocrit, hemoglobin, or lipid profile should be monitored at follow-up visits. Adequate levels of sex hormones are required to maintain bone mass; thus patients should avoid hypogonadism, particularly if they have undergone oophorectomy [12]. Otherwise, bone mineral density (BMD) screening can be initiated at age 60 or if testosterone levels are consistently low. Transgender men with cervixes and/or breast tissue should undergo age-appropriate cancer screening as indicated.

Testosterone therapy is contraindicated in patients who are pregnant and have unstable coronary artery disease, or untreated polycythemia (hematocrit at or above 55%). Testosterone therapy may exacerbate polycythemia and hyperlipidemia, which should be treated if present prior to introducing hormone therapies. It is unknown if testosterone therapy increases the risk for uterine or ovarian cancers. Currently there is insufficient evidence to recommend routine hysterectomy and/or oophorectomy in transgender men for the purpose of malignancy prevention.

Testosterone stimulates erythropoiesis; therefore transgender men should be monitored to ensure that hematocrit levels are less than 55% [12, 20].

General Health Surveillance and Screenings

The available data suggest that hormone therapy for transgender individuals is safe under clinician supervision [21]. Thrombogenic complications are a primary risk factor for transgender women who undergo feminizing hormone therapy [16]. Therefore, educating transgender women and their providers regarding preventative ways to minimize the risk of thromboembolic events might be the most important long-term intervention to minimize the risk of adverse effects from estrogen. Patients should be counseled to avoid smoking, a modifiable risk factor for venous thromboembolism. Although some advocate complete discontinuation of estrogen in transgender women with histories of thrombotic events, anti-coagulation regimens can be administered as needed in order to maintain the hormone treatment regimen while minimizing the risk of thromboembolism. Transgender women should also be monitored for hypertriglyceridemia and decreased libido, both of which commonly occur with feminizing hormone therapy [21].

It is well-established that androgens cause erythropoiesis stimulation [20]. Therefore, transgender men treated with testosterone should have their hematocrit checked regularly to exclude erythrocytosis. Dose adjustments and other interventions (e.g., phlebotomy) are sometimes required to achieve safe hematocrit levels [21].

Cancer screening of internal reproductive organs, such as the cervix, in transgender men is still necessary regardless of gender expression. Studies have suggested that testosterone therapy in transgender men results in atrophy of the cervical epithelium and endometrium. The corpus luteum may remain up to 1 year after the start of therapy [21]. Poorly powered studies have reported hyperplasia in ovarian stroma and ovarian cortex thickening in transgender men on testosterone therapy [21]. And although rare, breast cancer has been reported in transgender men [21]. For patients with retained breast tissue, routine mammography based on age should be encouraged per current guidelines [21].

Conclusions

Hormone therapy for transgender patients is safe when given by experienced providers in a monitored setting. Evidence of the effectiveness of hormone therapy can be seen in the dramatic rise of transgender patients seeking medical care [22]. Transgender patients are presenting to clinics for hormone therapy at younger ages and are less likely to acquire hormones from other sources. It is vital to mainstream transgender care among medical providers. Published transgender medical treatment guidelines provide a foundation for making transgender patient care more generalized and accessible to all healthcare providers.

References

1. Safer JD, Tangpricha V. Care of transgender persons. N Engl J Med. 2019;381(25):2451–60.
2. Safer JD, Pearce EN. A simple curriculum content change increased medical student comfort with transgender medicine. Endocr Pract. 2013;19(4):633–7.
3. Association AP. Diagnostic and statistical manual of mental disorders (DSM-5®). American Psychiatric Pub; 2013.

4. WHO Drops Being Transgender from List of Mental Disorders | Time. https://time.com/5596845/world-health-organization-transgender-identity/. Accessed 5 Apr 2021
5. Green R, Newman LE, Stoller RJ. Treatment of boyhood "transsexualism". Arch Gen Psychiatry. 1972;26(3):213–7.
6. Liao LM, et al. Determinant factors of gender identity: a commentary. J Pediatr Urol. 2012;8(6):597–601.
7. SOC V7_English.pdf. https://www.wpath.org/media/cms/Documents/SOC%20v7/SOC%20V7_English.pdf. Accessed 1 Apr 2021
8. Hembree WC, et al. Endocrine treatment of gender-dysphoric/gender-incongruent persons: an Endocrine Society clinical practice guideline. J Clin Endocrinol Metab. 2017;102(11):3869–903.
9. Wallien MS, Cohen-Kettenis PT. Psychosexual outcome of gender-dysphoric children. J Am Acad Child Adolesc Psychiatry. 2008;47(12):1413–23.
10. Cohen-Kettenis PT, Delemarre-van de Waal HA, Gooren LJ. The treatment of adolescent transsexuals: changing insights. J Sex Med. 2008;5(8):1892–7.
11. de Vries AL, et al. Puberty suppression in adolescents with gender identity disorder: a prospective follow-up study. J Sex Med. 2011;8(8):2276–83.
12. Hembree WC, et al. Endocrine treatment of transsexual persons: an Endocrine Society clinical practice guideline. J Clin Endocrinol Metab. 2009;94(9):3132–54.
13. Reisman T, Goldstein Z, Safer JD. A review of breast development in cisgender women and implications for transgender women. Endocr Pract. 2019;25(12):1338–45.
14. Nagarajan V, Chamsi-Pasha M, Tang WH. The role of aldosterone receptor antagonists in the management of heart failure: an update. Cleve Clin J Med. 2012;79(9):631–9.
15. Commissioner O of the FDA approves new oral testosterone capsule for treatment of men with certain forms of hypogonadism. FDA Published March 24, 2020. https://www.fda.gov/news-events/press-announcements/fda-approves-new-oral-testosterone-capsule-treatment-men-certain-forms-hypogonadism. Accessed 5 Apr 2021
16. Zucker R, Reisman T, Safer JD. Minimizing venous thromboembolism in feminizing hormone therapy: applying lessons from cisgender women and previous data. Endocr Pract. 2021;27(6):621–5.
17. Kozato A, et al. No venous thromboembolism increase among transgender female patients remaining on estrogen for gender-affirming surgery. J Clin Endocrinol Metab. 2021;106(4):e1586–90.
18. T'Sjoen G, et al. Endocrinology of transgender medicine. Endocr Rev. 2019;40(1):97–117.
19. Bockting W, Coleman E, De Cuypere G. Care of transsexual persons. N Engl J Med. 2011;364(26):2559–60. author reply 2560
20. Mullins ES, et al. Thrombosis risk in transgender adolescents receiving gender-affirming hormone therapy. Pediatrics. 2021.
21. Weinand JD, Safer JD. Hormone therapy in transgender adults is safe with provider supervision; a review of hormone therapy sequelae for transgender individuals. J Clin Transl Endocrinol. 2015;2(2):55–60.
22. Gardner IH, Safer JD. Progress on the road to better medical care for transgender patients. Curr Opin Endocrinol Diabetes Obes. 2013;20(6):553–8.

Chapter 3
Strategies for Evaluating Patients' Readiness for Surgical Intervention: From a Psychiatric Perspective

Max Lichtenstein

Behavioral and Surgical Treatment for Gender Dysphoria Due to Voice

Gender dysphoria is the distress one feels at the incongruence between their gender identity and the sex they were assigned at birth. Hormone therapy and gender-affirming surgeries help transgender individuals to align their primary and secondary sexual characteristics to better match their gender identity. Gender-affirming genital and chest/breast surgeries have long been shown to decrease gender dysphoria, improve the quality of life, and reduce psychiatric symptoms of transgender patients [1–4]. Procedures and surgeries addressing secondary sexual characteristics such as facial feminization [5], body contouring, and hair removal [6] have also been shown to reduce dysphoria and improve quality of life in these patients.

While the first surgery to change vocal pitch to a feminine range in natal males could be considered the Castrati of the 1500s, glottoplasty was not routinely preformed in transgender women until the 1980s. Even small studies on the effect and satisfaction of glottoplasty in transgender women were not done until the 2000s, and the topic remains understudied to this day. Vocal feminization has always been a treatment goal for transgender women, and advice on how to achieve feminine vocal cadence can be seen in the earliest publications by and for these women [7]. Voice reveals clues about the speaker's gender, age, emotion, and health through variations in pitch loudness and quality, and most listeners are able to intuit a person's gender through their speech patterns [8]. Transgender women are challenged daily to conform to feminine speech patterns in order to be identified as the correct gender. The latter presents obstacles for patients during phone or voice-only communication. Studies using patient satisfaction and quality-of-life scales have found

M. Lichtenstein (✉)
Department of Psychiatry, Icahn School of Medicine, New York, NY, USA
e-mail: max.lichtenstein@mountsinai.org

M. S. Courey et al. (eds.), *Voice and Communication in Transgender and Gender Diverse Individuals*, https://doi.org/10.1007/978-3-031-24632-6_3

Table 3.1 Gender-affirming procedures in transgender women in the United States [12]

Procedure	% who have had	% who want this	% who might want this	% who do not want this
Permanent hair removal	48	47	3	2
Voice therapy (non-surgical)	**14**	**48**	**17**	**21**
Vaginoplasty	12	54	22	12
Mammoplasty	11	40	30	19
Orchiectomy	11	47	22	20
Facial feminization	7	43	29	21
Tracheal shave	5	32	28	35
Silicone injections	3	10	27	60
Voice surgery	**1**	**18**	**32**	**49**
Others not listed procedure	6	15	15	64

vocal therapy with glottoplasty to significantly reduce this distress and improve quality of life related to voice [9–11].

The 2015 US Transgender Survey (USTS) [12] analyzed responses from over 30,000 transgender individuals in all US states and territories and found that vocal feminization was one of the most desired therapies among transgender women, where vocal surgery such as glottoplasty is less desired (Table 3.1). Both vocal therapy and glottoplasty had a large disparity between those who wanted the procedure and those who could access it.

Prohibitive cost and lack of insurance coverage are the biggest barriers to transgender people accessing gender-affirming glottoplasty. While considered medically necessary by national and international standards of care [13–15], insurance coverage for gender-affirming surgeries remains highly dependent on local anti-discrimination policy and healthcare coverage [16]. Coverage for surgery addressing secondary sexual characteristics is even sparser and for glottoplasty specifically is nearly nonexistent. An analysis of the top 3 commercial insurance carriers in all 50 states in the United States showed only 2.7% of carriers had a favorable policy on providing gender-affirming vocal interventions, with 75.8% providing no coverage and 13.4% having no policy [17].

The Role of a Pre-Surgical Psychiatric Assessment

The medical establishment has not been traditionally accepting of transgender people. Psychiatric gatekeeping has been a part of gender-affirming surgical assessment since standard-of-care guidelines have existed for such procedures. The first guidelines were published in 1969 by John Money and Robert Green [18]. These were modified by the Harry Benjamin International Gender Dysphoria Association (HBIGDA) in 1979 to create their first guidelines. The HBIGDA would later become the World Professional Association of Transgender Health (WPATH), the governing body that provides the standard-of-care guidelines most wildly used around the world today. Over time, the WPATH criteria have become less conservative, removing eligibility requirements for psychotherapy, narrow gender presentation, type of sexual activity, and the length of time recommended for hormone therapy and living in the desired gender role. The WPATH is now in its seventh edition of standard-of-care guidelines for medical treatment of gender dysphoria [14]. These guidelines recommend psychological assessment prior to surgery for genital (vaginoplasty, phalloplasty, etc.) and chest/breast surgeries. For other gender-affirming surgical procedures mentioned in the WPATH SoC 7 such as glottoplasty, facial feminization, body contouring, and chondrolaryngoplasty, no psychological assessment is recommended prior to performing these procedures. Other guidelines introduced more recently which emphasize surgical readiness, like the Gender ASSET and Mount Sinai Patient-Centered Pre-surgical Care Model, also do not recommend routine psychological assessment prior to glottoplasty [19, 20].

Despite the clear recommendation that no psychological assessment is required for glottoplasty, in the United States, insurance companies and Medicare/Medicaid require "letters of support" from mental health providers in order to cover the procedure. The most commonly used criteria for those insurance providers that cover surgery at all are adopted from the WPATH guidelines for gender-affirming genital and chest/breast surgeries. These letters must be written by a psychiatrist, psychologist (PhD or PsyD), psychiatric nurse practitioner, or licensed clinical social worker (LCSW). Some plans demand an additional letter from a physician with an ongoing relationship with the patient or a letter from a doctorate-level mental health provider, which further limits access to care. This task is often difficult given the shortage of mental health providers across the country [21] and even fewer with knowledge of transgender medicine [22]. There is no evidence that these assessments benefit the patient or prevent unnecessary surgery.

The recommendation of the author of this chapter and book editors is that no psychiatric assessment is needed prior to transgender individuals seeking glottoplasty. We also understand that most patients are required to complete these assessments in order for benefits to cover this procedure.

Conducting a Pre-Surgical Psychiatric Assessment

Once the number and qualification of the writer of letters has been established by the benefits provider, the psychiatric assessment for gender-affirming surgeries is straightforward and contains four parts. A diagnostic assessment of gender dysphoria, a gender history that includes length of time living as their gender role and time on hormone therapy, a general psychiatric diagnostic and risk assessment and a capacity assessment.

First, the mental health practitioner must establish a diagnosis of gender dysphoria as per the DSM5 [23] (Table 3.2). The informed patient will meet many of these

Table 3.2 Diagnosing gender dysphoria in adults and adolescents

A. A marked incongruence between one's experienced/expressed gender and assigned gender for at least 6 months' duration, as manifested by at least two of the following:
1. A marked incongruence between one's experienced/expressed gender and the primary and/or secondary sex characteristics (or in young adolescents, anticipated secondary sex characteristics)
2. A strong desire to be rid of one's primary and/or secondary sex characteristics because of a marked incongruence between of a marked incongruence with ones experienced expressed gender (or in young adolescents a desire to prevent the development of anticipated secondary sex characteristics)
3. A strong desire for the primary and/or secondary sex characteristics of the other gender
4. A strong desire to be of the other gender (or some alternative gender different from ones assigned gender)
5. A strong desire to be treated of the other gender (or some alternative gender different from ones assigned gender)
6. A strong conviction the one has the typical feelings and reactions of the other gender (or some alternative gender different from ones assigned gender)
B. The condition is associated with clinically significant distress in impairment in social, occupational, or other important areas of functioning

criteria simply by seeking glottoplasty. It is not the clinician's duty to determine the "correct" gender of the patient, but rather if glottoplasty will improve dysfunction caused by gender dysphoria. The vocal surgeon can provide objective assessment of the vocal pitch, and the mental health provider should focus on the subjective distress the patient has from their voice. The clinician should ask how the patient's voice impacts their life in interpersonal, professional, and day-to-day settings. Many transgender individuals find that misgendering (being identified as the wrong gender) is particularly painful or common over the phone or when seeking or providing customer service. The clinician should also ask if less invasive measures have been taken such as vocal therapy (professional or self-help) and what effects these have had on the patient's dysphoria.

Second, the clinician will conduct a simple gender history. The interview should always begin by asking the patient the gender they identify with now and what gender was on their birth certificate. The clinician should then offer their own pronouns when asking the patient which ones they use (e.g., "Hello, I am Dr. Smith and I use she/her pronouns, which pronouns may I use when speaking about you?"). Starting with open-ended questions, the clinician may begin by asking when the patient first began to feel different from the gender they were assigned at birth. Let the patient lead the discussion to other important events in their transition. Puberty, discovering other transgender people, coming out to loved ones, starting to live as their gender role in public, and starting on hormone therapy are often significant events. A detailed gender history is not necessary for pre-surgical assessment unless the patient plans to engage in longer-term therapy with the provider. Collecting the length of time the patient has been on hormone therapy and the length of time living in their desired gender role is adequate.

WPATH guidelines recommend that the hormone therapy be provided by a clinician for greater than 12 months; however many transgender people do not have access to adequate transgender medical care so seek treatment from non-clinicians or more recently from Internet pharmacies. The clinician may use their own judgment if the patient has been in consistent and adequate care if the patient is not getting hormone therapy from a licensed clinical provider. Feminizing hormone therapy may not be indicated for patients for many reasons including medical contraindications such as increased risk of blood clotting, side effects such as sexual dysfunction, or because the patient does not desire the effects of hormone therapy as part of their transition such as breast growth. Referring patients to adequate care if they have not been on adequately administered or desired hormone therapy should be provided if necessary.

The 12-month requirement living in the desired gender role is meant to allow time for adjustment to then often profound challenges in vocational, interpersonal, legal, and economic areas of life transgender people frequently face when first transitioning before undergoing irreversible surgery. This requirement is based on genital surgeries, not glottoplasty, and may not be generalizable to this procedure. This is often called the "living full time" requirement, as it mandates the patient present in their desired gender role consistently in day-to-day life. This requires coming out in all areas of life: to family, employers, and members of their community. This is often a tumultuous time in a transgender person's life, and gender-affirming therapy or counseling can be recommended during this time. Counseling is no longer recommended for every patient seeking surgery and should be sought at the patient's discretion.

Third, the clinician should do a general psychiatric diagnostic assessment with risk assessment. Areas covered should include presence and history of mood, personality, anxiety, trauma-related, psychotic, eating, and developmental disorders. The patient's current psychiatric treatment and treatment history including medications, therapy, hospitalizations, and major psychiatric episodes should be recorded. Substance use including nicotine should be assessed and independently evaluated via urine or serum toxicology at the clinician's discretion. A risk assessment should be made based on if the patient's current psychiatric state will impair their surgical outcome. This should be a high bar to delay surgery, and there are no mental health conditions that are absolute contraindications to gender-affirming surgery. Acute psychotic or manic episodes should be treated and resolved before the patient undergoes any type of surgery. A general recommendation of 6 months of recovery following psychiatric hospitalization before undergoing surgery can be followed. More chronic symptoms of personality, obsessive compulsive, eating, post-traumatic stress, depressive, and anxiety disorders should be evaluated and assessed in relation to their impact on the patient's expected surgical recovery. Suicidal ideation alone is not a surgical contraindication and is unfortunately epidemic in the transgender population [12, 24, 25]. If the patient is acutely suicidal, then their safety should be the first priority and managed in acute care setting, with discussion of surgery tabled until they are no longer in imminent danger. Gender-affirming surgeries improve psychiatric outcomes and suicidal ideation in these same patients and so can be part of a treatment plan for gender dysphoria.

Psychiatric contraindications to surgery are extremely rare and usually readily evident. Examples may include depression that severely impacts a patient's hygiene, an active substance use disorder, agoraphobia preventing a patient from getting adequate follow-up, or psychosis that would impact the patients understanding of the surgery and recovery. In cases such as these psychiatric and/or other mental health services should be offered.

Lastly, the patient must have the capacity to consent to treatment and be of consenting age in the jurisdiction where the surgery is taking place (generally 18 years old). A capacity assessment assesses four parts of a patient's understanding when making a medical decision; their ability to make a choice, their understanding of the risks and benefits of the procedure, their appreciation of those risks and benefits, and the logical reasoning used to make the decision. A patient must be able to state a clear and consistent choice in their medical decision, choosing glottoplasty over vocal therapy or no treatment. If the patient is unaware of other choices, then the clinician should provide information and assess how and why that impacts their decision. The patient must be familiar with the risk and desired outcomes of glottoplasty. If they have not yet met with a surgeon, the clinician must be informed enough about the medical procedure sought to provide some general education about the expected outcomes and high-risk complications. The patients should be able to absorb this information into their decision-making process and be able to apply these facts their own circumstances. The ability to appreciate risks refers to one's ability to recognize how facts are relevant to themselves. Dismissal of medical complications due to poor insight or delusional beliefs may result in lack of capacity. Lastly, the patient must come to their conclusion based on logical reasoning which will draw on a patient's own beliefs and values. Patients who are unable to incorporate new information or rely on a delusional belief system would lack capacity. Clinicians unfamiliar with capacity assessments may use the following table (Table 3.3) to help assess the capacity to consent to glottoplasty specifically.

Table 3.3 A guide to help assess a patient's decision-making capacity

Decision-making ability	Definition	Sample questions
Consistent choice	Ability to state a clear decision	"Based on what you know about vocal feminization, what options are available?" "What options have you chosen?"
Understanding risks and outcomes	Ability to state the meaning of relevant information (e.g., risks/benefits, procedure, recovery time)	After giving the patient information, ask "in your own words, can you tell me what I said about what happens during glottoplasty?/What risks are there?/What is the recovery like?"
Appreciation of risks and outcomes	Ability to explain how information applies to oneself	To assess appreciation of risk, "Do you think there is a possibility the surgery can harm you?" To assess appreciation of outcomes, "What are you hoping the surgery will do to your voice? What will it not be able to do to your voice?"
Reasoning	Ability to compare information and infer consequences of choices	To assess comparative reasoning, "How is glottoplasty better than vocal therapy alone for you?" To assess consequential reasoning, "How could having glottoplasty affect your everyday life?" "What would you do if you had "complication X" from the surgery?"

Conclusion

Achieving a feminine vocal perception improves quality of life and reduces gender dysphoria and associated psychiatric symptoms in transgender women. Glottoplasty is a medically necessary surgery for those for whom less invasive vocal therapies have been inadequate. No routine psychiatric evaluation is recommended for patients seeking glottoplasty, though benefits providers who cover the surgery in the United States will still require them. Psychiatric evaluation for genital surgery as per the WPATH standards of care is usually inappropriately applied to glottoplasty. These psychiatric evaluations must establish the capacity to consent to the procedure, a diagnosis of gender dysphoria as per the DSM-V, 12 months taking continuous hormone therapy, and living in the desired gender role and that severe psychiatric symptoms are well controlled enough for the patient to undergo surgery and safe recovery.

References

1. Nobili A, Glazebrook C, Arcelus J. Quality of life of treatment-seeking transgender adults: a systematic review and meta-analysis. Rev Endocr Metab Disord. 2018;19(3):199–220.
2. Johansson A, Sundbom E, Höjerback T, Bodlund O. A five-year follow-up study of Swedish adults with gender identity disorder. Arch Sex Behav. 2010;39(6):1429–37.
3. Weigert R, Frison E, Sessiecq Q, Al Mutairi K, Casoli V. Patient satisfaction with breasts and psychosocial, sexual, and physical well-being after breast augmentation in male-to-female transsexuals. Plast Reconstr Surg. 2013;132:1421–9.
4. De Cuypere G, T'Sjoen G, Beerten R, et al. Sexual and physical health after sex reassignment surgery. Arch Sex Behav. 2005;34:679–90.
5. Ainsworth TA, Spiegel JH. quality of life of individuals with and without facial feminization surgery or gender reassignment surgery. Qual Life Res. 2010;19:1019–24.
6. Bradford NJ, Rider GN, Spencer KG. Hair removal and psychological well-being in trans-feminine adults: associations with gender dysphoria and gender euphoria. J Dermatolog Treat. 2021;32(6):635–42.
7. Prince V. Transvestia archive at the university of Victoria. 1960-1986. https://vault.library.uvic.ca/collections/6576cedf-1282-4089-8351-08f73f4199b4
8. Gallena SJK, Stickels B, Stickels E. Gender perception after raising vowel fundamental and formant frequencies: considerations for oral resonance research. J Voice. 2018;32:592–601.
9. Brown SK, Chang J, Hu S, Sivakumar G, Sataluri M, Goldberg L, Courey MS. Addition of Wendler Glottoplasty to voice therapy improves trans female voice outcomes. Laryngoscope. 2021;131(7):1588–93.
10. Gray ML, Courey MS. Transgender voice and communication. Otolaryngol Clin N Am. 2019;52(4):713–22.
11. Casado JC, Rodríguez-Parra MJ, Adrián JA. Voice feminization in male-to-female transgendered clients after Wendler's glottoplasty with vs. without voice therapy support. Eur Arch Otorhinolaryngol. 2017;274(4):2049–58.
12. James S, Herman J, Rankin S, et al. US transgender survey report on health and healthcare, vol. 2016. Washington, DC: National Center for Transgender Equality; 2015.
13. Etner R, Monstrey S, Coleman E. Principles of transgender medicine and surgery. 2nd ed. New York, NY: Routledge; 2016.
14. World Professional Association for Transgender Health. Standards of Care for Transsexual, Transgender, and Gender Nonconforming People, Version 7. Published 2011.
15. Hembree WC, Cohen-Kettenis PT, Gooren L, Hannema SE, Meyer WJ, Hassan Murad M, Rosenthal SM, Safer JD, Tangpricha V, T'Sjoen GG. Endocrine treatment of gender-dysphoric/gender-incongruent persons: an Endocrine Society clinical practice guideline. J Clin Endocrinol Metabol. 2017;102(11):3869–903.
16. Thoreson N, Marks DH, Peebles JK, King DS, Dommasch E. Health insurance coverage of permanent hair removal in transgender and gender-minority patients. JAMA Dermatol. 2020;156(5):561–5.
17. DeVore EK, Gadkaree SK, Richburg K, Banaszak EM, Wang TV, Naunheim MR, Shaye DA. Coverage for gender-affirming voice surgery and therapy for transgender individuals. Laryngoscope. 2021;131(3):E896–902. https://doi.org/10.1002/lary.28986. Epub 2020 Aug 10
18. Green R, Money J. Transsexualism and sex reassignment. Baltimore, MD: The Johns Hopkins Press; 1969.
19. Lichtenstein M, Stein L, Connolly E, Goldstein ZG, Martinson T, Tiersten L, Shin SJ, Pang JH, Safer JD. The Mount Sinai Patient-Centered Preoperative Criteria Meant to Optimize Outcomes Are Less of a Barrier to Care Than WPATH SOC 7 Criteria Before Transgender-Specific Surgery. Transgend Health. 2020;5(3):166–72. https://doi.org/10.1089/trgh.2019.0066. PMID: 33644310; PMCID: PMC7906222.
20. Keo-Meier K, Keo-Meier B. The Gender ASSET: Gender Affirmative Supportive Surgery Tool. https://gendereducationnetwork.com/courses/thegenderasset/

21. Olfson M. Building the mental health workforce capacity needed to treat adults with serious mental illnesses. Health Aff (Millwood). 2016;35(6):983–90.
22. Korpaisarn S, Safer JD. Gaps in transgender medical education among healthcare providers: a major barrier to care for transgender persons. Rev Endocr Metab Disord. 2018;19(3):271–5.
23. American Psychiatric Association. Diagnostic and statistical manual of mental disorders. 5th ed. Arlington, VA: American Psychiatric Association; 2013.
24. Narang P, Sarai SK, Aldrin S, Lippmann S. Suicide among transgender and gender-nonconforming people. Prim Care Companion CNS Disord. 2018;20(3):26899.
25. Wolford-Clevenger C, Cannon CJ, Flores LY, Smith PN, Stuart GL. Suicide risk among transgender people: a prevalent problem in critical need of empirical and theoretical research. Violence Gend. 2017;4(3):69–72.

Chapter 4
Barriers to Care and Cultural Responsiveness in Transgender and Gender Nonconforming Voice Modification

A. C. Goldberg and Ruchi Kapila

Introduction

You enter a crowded clinic waiting room and check in. You give the name you used when registering in the online portal. The front desk staff hands you some paperwork. You stare blankly, not knowing what name to write on the top line of the form. You decide not to ask at the desk and list your deadname first with your real name in quotation marks. Then...the questions. The boxes. The M/F. The "other." The surgical history. The "other professionals we may contact" list. It's all so triggering. You sit surrounded by pride flags and safe space stickers feeling irritated and unseen. You turn in your paperwork and wait anxiously. You hear whispering. The front desk staff and the clinician are talking about your name. What will they say out loud when they call you? You look around at others and wonder what they'll think if your deadname is called out. Is it safe? The clinician opens the door with your paperwork in hand, and your heart is pounding.

The experience described above is almost universal to transgender and gender nonconforming (TGNC) people in clinical settings. This chapter will deconstruct and reframe constructs to help readers identify and address issues within their settings in order to increase their cultural responsiveness.

Anyone of any gender or gender presentation may seek the services or procedures discussed throughout this chapter; this includes cisgender people. That is to say the label "transgender female" or "female" to describe people or voices will not be used. If a nonbinary person who feels their resonance is too chesty or their pitch too low came to seek these services, assuming their process as "feminization" would

A. C. Goldberg (✉)
Transplaining LLC, Massachusetts Public Schools, The CREDITs Institute, Cambridge, MA, USA

R. Kapila
Kapila Voice and Speech Services, Hayward, CA, USA

M. S. Courey et al. (eds.), *Voice and Communication in Transgender and Gender Diverse Individuals*, https://doi.org/10.1007/978-3-031-24632-6_4

be a misnomer, as well as a *microaggression*, a statement, act, or episode that (un) intentionally or incidentally highlights prejudice or bias toward a minoritized person or group. As a clinician, using terminology that fits is critical to the therapeutic relationship. The assumption that someone wants a certain vocal presentation because of their gender is a slippery slope that clinicians must approach through a culturally responsive lens.

Further, language is dynamic and changes over time. Terms used in this chapter may be outdated by the time of publication. Please see sources for up-to-date terminology around the TGNC population and services. Remember, clients will describe themselves, follow their lead.

Language

In order to engage in culturally responsive practices, it is crucial to understand and use the same terms that clients use to describe themselves. Definitions of some general terms as they relate to identities and voice care are listed below. An all-inclusive list of gender terminology cannot exist given the constantly evolving definitions, titles, labels, and terms within TGNC communities, and any list of TGNC-related terms must be routinely updated (Table 4.1). The use of language (and avoidance of terms) should be led by and agreed to by the client. Refer to "The Trans Language Primer" (available at https://www.translanguageprimer.org/); Parents, Families, and Friends of Lesbians and Gays (PFLAG) National Glossary of Terms (available on https://pflag.org/glossary); and Gender Minorities' "Trans 101: glossary of trans words and how to use them" (available on https://genderminorities.com/database/glossary-transgender/).

Below are some initial terms that often arise in the TGNC community:

Transgender person: A person whose sense of gender differs from the societal expectations placed on them based on their sex assigned at birth.

Table 4.1 Examples of current and outdated terminology as of May 2021. Caveat: List is not inclusive of current and outdated terminology

Current/neutral terms	Outdated or loaded/biased terms
• Transgender (transgender man, transgender woman) • Nonbinary/enby • Transmasculine • Transfeminine • Two-spirit/2S • Genderqueer • Genderfluid • Flux • Bigender • Pangender • Cisgender	• Transsexual • Transgendered • Gender identity • Gender dysphoria • Passing • Biological sex • Identifies as • Real name • Preferred pronouns

Nonbinary person: A person whose gender is neither male nor female. Male/female may be characteristics within a nonbinary gender or may not even be relevant. A nonbinary gender cannot be neatly defined, as gender is an experience that varies from person to person.

Genderfluid person: A person whose gender is not set at a fixed point and may vary from day to day.

Genderqueer person: A person whose gender does not fit squarely into a box and may or may not vary from day to day.

Cisgender person: A person whose sense of gender aligns with society's expectations placed on them based on their sex assigned at birth.

Asking someone's gender identity is irrelevant unless the client asserts otherwise. In any setting, the most important things to know about clients are their *names*, *pronouns*, and *goals*. Not everyone who presents for "transfeminine" voice care wants their voice to sound the same. Some clients may bring up "passing" or being *cis-assumed*. The term "passing" should be avoided unless this is reflecting the client's language, as it is a loaded term and a construct many transgender people wish to dismantle. "Cis-assumed" puts the onus on the observer for assuming gender identity and does not imbue the transgender individual with a value as compared to cisgender norms.

What Is "Voice Feminization"?

"Voice feminization" does not have a monolithic definition. Gender identity or many other additional identities based on appearance and voice alone cannot be assumed. Pertinent information in holistically supporting a client's identity involves careful and trauma-informed care approach in intake. Standards and goals for "voice feminization" may be cisgender-clinician led or established, which may not be representative of the goals of the transgender woman, nonbinary, or transfeminine client. When discussing presumably cisgender women's voices, there is a wide variety in pitch, resonance, and vocal tract configurations. Thus, "voice feminization" should be framed from the values and perspectives of the client to set appropriate goals and demystify the acoustic and auditory perceptual markers by which to determine progress. Through this investigation and deconstruction, terms that are clinical, inclusive, and more client-centered can be identified and used.

If a client requests voice services and says they want a "more feminine" vocal presentation, the best practices should include:

1. *Asking what the client would like their voice to sound like and examples of voices they enjoy hearing.* Although a client may use certain pronouns, this does not mean they want to conform to stereotypical or binary gender norms. Always ask for clarification and direct attention to the client's preferences and perspectives (e.g., "Whose voice do you like listening to?", "What kinds of voices are you drawn to?", "What do you enjoy about your voice and what do you wish to

change?"). Listen to and discuss varied vocal presentations with the client, acknowledging that voices are as diverse as all the gender presentations that exist.
2. *Taking gendered terminology out of describing voice targets, unless specified by the client, and reflecting language used by the client.* Use clinical, unbiased language after providing education and demonstrating vocal targets to support your client's comprehension and generalization (e.g., "For this vocal presentation, the focus can be on more forward resonance.").
3. *Checking in about the client's experience when attempting voice modifications or techniques – focusing on the client's response to how something sounds or feels, rather than instrumental data.* Consent-driven care (discussed further in this chapter) requires the focus to be on the client's perspectives as well as a sense of safety and affirmation instead of asserting the clinician's vocal targets. Inquiring and emphasizing the client's experience and perspectives not only facilitate trust and rapport but also ensure the efficacy of intervention by clarifying whether goals are being addressed per the client.

Brief Historical Considerations for the Transgender and Gender Nonconforming Community in the United States

TGNC communities use myriad language to describe identities and experiences across international communities. Describing historical considerations for an underrepresented and, at many times, oppressed community with traditionally academic sources is a challenge given the often limited support and funding for preserving their histories. With the understanding that this chapter cannot encapsulate all global gender-expansive communities and their nuances, it will provide a brief historical foundation regarding transgender communities in the United States and considerations for voice services and interventions provided within this community.

Before assertions of "transsexual [identity]" in the 1960s and 1970s, which morphed and expanded to "transgender" in the 1980s and 1990s, multilayered examples of gender variation were also present in the early nineteenth and twentieth centuries [1]. This spans back to indigenous two-spirit people of this nation (formerly referred to as "berdaches") who asserted many different, native names and were found across nearly 160 tribes. Considered to inhabit a third or fourth gender, these people combined gender roles and clothing presentation, but "historical analysis...is difficult, given the layered interpretations of both colonial record-keepers... and modern-day, queer Native American observers" [1].

Service Providers

In 2011, the World Professional Association for Transgender Health (WPATH) included voice and communication intervention in the Standards of Care version 7 (SOC 7) and added speech and voice (now voice and communication) to their list of treatments. While this publication is encompassing of the interventions and considerations carried out by speech-language pathologies (SLPs) for gender-affirming voice considerations, there is little discussion of the impact of voice workers and professionals within and ancillary to the community for these voice modifications. Per Kozan and Hammond [2] in "The Singing Voice," WPATH asserts in SOC 7 that other voice professionals play a "valuable adjunct role" but that SLPs are the primary providers of service. Although there is value in interdisciplinary accountability, there is a greater need for accountability to TGNC leaders irrespective of background, to ensure transparency and an archival history of gender-affirming voice modification from community perspectives. Voice and communication modification services for the TGNC community are not "therapy" unless an underlying vocal pathology, a medical diagnosis, or a deficit in cognitive communication, speech, or language is present. If these services are provided in the absence of vocal, medical, or communicative compromise, then they are considered habilitative in which case singing voice specialists, voice coaches, diction coaches, theatre voice professionals, and others with sufficient cultural responsiveness and vocal training may provide these services. Equitable collaboration with TGNC individuals will facilitate the intention to advocate for and establish interdisciplinary, interconnected community-based cultural responsiveness accountability.

Discrimination in Healthcare and Disparities in Health Outcomes in TGNC Community

Research, in brief, according to the National Center for Transgender Equality (2018)

Health outcomes for all categories of respondents show the negative effects of social and economic marginalization.

Refusal of care: *Nineteen percent (19%) of the sample reported refusal of medical care* due to their transgender or gender nonconforming status, with even higher numbers among people of color in the survey.

Uninformed doctors: *Fifty percent (50%) of the sample reported having to teach their medical providers* about TGNC care.

Postponed care: Survey participants reported that when they were sick or injured, *many postponed medical care due to discrimination (28%)* or inability to afford it (48%).

Medical records not representative of gender identity: Of those who have transitioned gender, *only one-fifth (21%) have been able to update all of their identifications (IDs) and records with their new gender.* One-third (33%) of those who had transitioned had updated *none* of their IDs/records.

Lack of access to representative forms of identification: Only 59% reported updating the gender on their driver's license/state ID, meaning *41% live without ID that matches their gender identity.*

Violence in response to presenting non-representative forms of identification: *Forty percent (40%) of those who presented ID* (when it was required in the ordinary course of life) that did not match their gender identity/expression *reported being* *harassed, 3% reported being attacked or assaulted*, and 15% reported being asked to leave.

The aforementioned data is from the 2018 National Center for Transgender Equality's full report. When practicing through a trauma-informed lens, it is essential to acknowledge this data: if 50% of all TGNC people report having to educate providers, there is a greater likelihood that transgender patients and clients will not trust cisgender providers unless they create a space in which TGNC community members feel safe. Many TGNC people report being turned away from medical services, not only because of their gender presentations but also due to lack of identification (ID) that matches a current name and gender presentation. The trauma resulting from refusal to provide routine medical care due to incongruences with government ID and insurance (which is out of the control of the TGNC individual) is not something easily remedied. Given inadequate support and advocacy, these barriers to medical intervention are ongoing and a daily challenge for many TGNC people [3].

International and Domestic Studies Establish a Trend: *Despite Growing Awareness of TGNC Community, Cultural Responsiveness Training Is Largely Unchanged and Not Sought Out by Providers*

In Australia, numerous studies demonstrate that concern over using incorrect terminology or accidentally offending patients keeps providers from seeking education and engaging in culturally responsive practices [4]. Since 2000, evidence that this applies to service provision in the United States remains unchanged as of the publication of this 2015 review. Since 2007, the most commonly reported barrier to care is lack of access to TGNC-friendly providers. "Despite the growing evidence supporting the value of treating transgender patients in a mindful, supportive setting, the transgender health curriculum in most provider curricula remains unchanged" [5].

When surveyed, TGNC people report that language is one of the explicit markers in identifying if a space is safe to seek care. This issue is cyclical and will not resolve unless providers are committed to learning continually.

When this data is considered in the context of speech-language pathology, a 2019 brief survey (pending publication) revealed 86% of SLP respondents reported having received no formal training for working with TGNC patients, clients, and students. Eight percent (8%) reported receiving training but only with regard to voice services. No respondents stated that they underwent "general" cultural responsiveness training regarding TGNC individuals, and 6% were "unsure" about received training. This is an omission of essential education in the SLP field for a growing, marginalized, and vulnerable population.

Trauma-Informed Practice with TGNC Individuals

Trauma-informed care should be employed for all communities, even outside of TGNC populations and gender voice modification considerations. When working with TGNC individuals, it is more likely that they have experienced trauma in their lives. The focus of this approach is not to treat the trauma itself, but to cultivate and employ a holistic lens that centers the individual and their life experiences, with the goal of preventing re-traumatization and avoiding potential triggers. The TGNC population frequently experiences and processes these triggers as a form of anti-transgender bias.

The negative impact of anti-transgender bias on the mental health of TGNC people is currently explored through Hendricks and Testa's [6] adaptation of *the minority stress model* [7]. Anti-transgender bias, if experienced as an external event, is conceptualized as *distal minority stress*. Hendricks and Testa [6] defined four types of distal minority stressors for transgender people: *gender-related discrimination*, *gender-related rejection*, *gender-related victimization*, and *gender-related non-affirmation*. These stressors lead to increased psychological distress and increased individual experiences of internal or more proximal minority stressors [7]. Proximal minority stressors for transgender people, as defined by Hendricks and Testa [6], include *internalized transphobia*, *expectation of discrimination and rejection in future events*, and *nondisclosure (or concealment of transgender identity or history)*. The minority stress model theorizes that proximal minority stressors partially inform the relationship between distal minority stressors and mental health outcomes [6, 7]. Research documenting a relationship between transgender-specific proximal stressors and psychological distress has provided support for this theory and its application [8]. Thus, reducing all distal minority stressors in healthcare settings would decrease incidences of proximal minority stressors and is vital for the health and well-being of the TGNC community at large.

The *five principles of trauma-informed care* (or *TIC*, Fig. 4.1), provide an introductory model to preventing re-traumatization of vulnerable communities, including TGNC people, in the contexts of clinical and holistic care settings [9].

Safety
Choice
Collaboration
Trustworthiness
Empowerment
Definitions
Ensuring physical and emotional safety
Individual has choice and control
Making decisions with the individual and sharing power
Task clarity, consistency, and Interpersonal Boundaries
Prioritizing empowerment and skill building
Principles in Practice
Common areas are welcoming and privacy is respected
Individuals are provided a clear and appropriate message about their rights and responsibilities
Individuals are provided a significant role in planning and evaluating services
Respectful and professional boundaries are maintained
Providing an atmosphere that allows individuals to feel validated and affirmed with each and every contact at the agency

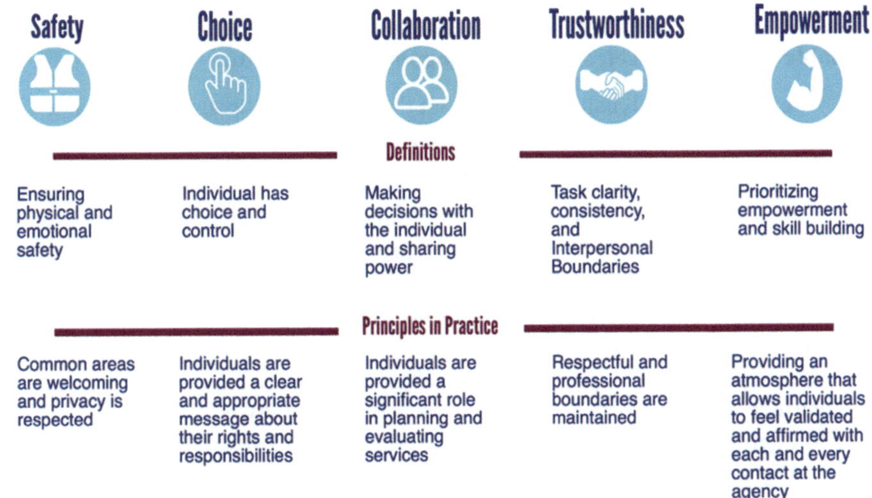

Fig. 4.1 The five principles of trauma-informed care

Adapting TIC Considerations to Institutional Settings [10, 11]

1. **Affirming the patient's gender throughout the encounter, from institution to interaction.**
   - Train front desk staff, anyone who answers phones and anyone who may have contact with the client within the entire institution. No one should be greeted with a binary honorific (miss/sir) and instead should be addressed in an inclusive manner at all times ("how can I help you today?").
   - Follow up with clients to assure they have been treated respectfully throughout their experience. A safe option may be a survey taken online, so that the patient feels comfortable giving honest feedback.
2. **Performing any physical exam in a collaborative manner that resists re-traumatization.**
   - Get consent for each component of examination, and talk the patient through it. "May I put my hand on the front of your neck?" "I'm going to use a light and tongue depressor to screen your oral cavity, is that ok?" "Tell me if any of this makes you uncomfortable."
   - Collaborate. "If you feel comfortable, you can put my fingers where you feel the pain or point it out for me. What works better for you?"
   - Recognize symptoms and findings that may suggest a history of trauma.
3. **Obtaining the history in a patient-led manner.**
   - Ask about trauma (only if clinically relevant) in a manner that resists re-traumatization.
   - Recognize and respond productively when a client becomes triggered.
   - Respond appropriately to trauma disclosure.
   - Follow "Do's and Don'ts" of intake (see below).
4. **Collaboratively creating care plans that are patient- empowering and enable mutual respect, safety, and ongoing engagement.**
   - Attend to power dynamics throughout the encounter: "Is this comfortable for you?" "Only share what you feel safe sharing."
   - "Please let me know if anything I say or do lands in the wrong way." "I want to make sure you feel safe and comfortable coming back to us: do you have any feedback? This is a collaborative process, and there is no time limit on providing feedback."
   - Facilitate connection to TGNC-specific, trauma support services if necessary to refer (e.g., mental health counselor, social worker, primary care physician (PCP), psychologist, peer support groups).
   - Partner with the client to determine their treatment goals.
   - Recognize, celebrate, and build on the client's strengths over time – employ a strength-based, dynamic, and functional model to ensure client agency and empowerment.

5. **Creating intake forms that can be filled out by anyone comfortably.**
    - "Name we should call you in clinic" should be at the top of your forms.
    - "Pronouns" should follow.
    - If legal name or gender marker information is required for insurance purposes, simply ask to obtain a copy of the client's driver's license when they turn in their forms.
    - Do not ask about marital status. Ask instead: "Do you live alone?" or "Do you have a healthcare proxy?"
    - Ask explicit permission for an emergency contact and verify which name(s) and pronouns are used with this person.
6. **Cultivating a safe and comfortable common area or waiting room.**
    - If you do not know what name to call someone aloud, just say their last name without an honorific (e.g., "Last Name: Smith").
    - Have all-gender restrooms, no matter what.
    - Keep rest room keys in an accessible space at the front desk.
    - Instruct front desk staff not to question clients aloud in the waiting area, and identify "confidential" spaces for interview.
    - Only have flags and "safe space" signs if every other suggestion on this list is followed and there is a commitment to continuing education on *TIC* for minoritized populations.

TIC also involves limiting interview questions to what is pertinent in care and/or service provision without asking for highly personal and/or triggering information. Below are some suggestions for TIC-based consensual intake and interview protocol.

Consent

When approaching treatment from a *TIC* lens, consent is one of the most important aspects of building a trust in a clinical relationship. Some clinicians tend to think of consent in terms of documentation, institutional liability, or physical contact with the client. Consent is for all interactions – physical, verbal (including communication with other providers), written (including documentation and email), and electronic medical records (Table 4.2).

Broadly, there are four types of consent that apply to clinical situations [12]:

1. *Implied:* a client answers questions without any objection.
2. *Expressed* (broadly defined): a client has signed a form saying they consent to treatment or has entered a room, willingly, with a clinician/provider.
3. *Documented:* a client has signed a front desk form.

Table 4.2 "Do's and don'ts" of intake/interview

Do	Don't	Rationale
Ask about pronouns	Ask about gender	You cannot tell a person's pronouns by knowing their gender
Ask about surgeries related to head, neck, heart, brain, face, voice, respiratory status, and intubation history	Ask for open-ended surgical history	This is a sensitive topic for TGNC people—Stick to what is clinically relevant
Ask about how often the client will be able to use their "new habitual/new target" voice	Ask invasive questions (e.g., "When did you come out?" "Are you fully out?" "When did you start transitioning?")	This can be a sensitive topic and a matter of personal and professional safety for many TGNC people. It is not clinically relevant to know that someone is not "out" to certain community members (e.g., their family if they only visit once a year). The focus should be on how often someone is able to use their new habitual voice
Ask about support network	Ask about "family support"	Many TGNC people do not have traditional family support and may rely on friends and community members instead. Reinforcing the lack of family support can impact trust and rapport in the service provision relationship

4. *Informed*: provider has fully explained process/procedure to client, client has the capacity to accept or decline, and client understands their privacy rights with regard to all interactions, including risks and disclosure of sensitive information.

Informed consent is the gold standard of consent and is *not a one-time conversation* about the outcome and potential risks of treatment. Throughout the course of treatment, even within each session, consent should be discussed through every interaction.

Consent throughout every interaction can be bridged in these ways:

"Can I ask you some questions?"
"Will you tell me if any of this makes you uncomfortable?"
"How do you like to receive feedback?"
"Do you want my feedback?" (before/after cueing).
"Who can I use this name and pronoun with?"

"Informed consent has become the primary paradigm for protecting the legal rights of clients and guiding the ethical practice of medicine. It may be used for different purposes in different contexts: legal, ethical or administrative. Although these purposes overlap, they are not identical, thus leading to different standards and criteria for what constitutes "adequate" informed consent" [13].

SLPs use informed consent for all of these purposes. The American Speech-Language-Hearing Association (ASHA) asserts informed consent "[m]ay be verbal, unless written consent is required; constitutes consent by persons served, research participants engaged, or parents and/or guardians of persons served to a proposed course of action after the communication of adequate information regarding expected outcomes and potential risks." It delineates in Principle of Ethics I, Part H that "[i]ndividuals [SLPs] shall obtain informed consent from the persons they serve about the nature and possible risks and effects of services provided, technology employed, and products dispensed" and "[t]his obligation also includes informing persons served about possible effects of not engaging in treatment or not following clinical recommendations [and i]f diminished decision-making ability of persons served is suspected, individuals should seek appropriate authorization for services, such as authorization from a spouse, other family member, or legally authorized/appointed representative [14]."

Given the assertion that goal setting and voice service provision is client-led and client-directed in gender-affirming voice, informed consent is paramount to ensuring affirmation, safety, and quality in services provided. Clients must be informed of their agency in this clinician-client relationship to determine goals and advocate for their right to navigate and use voice interventions as they see fit to achieve personal satisfaction in their vocal presentation, *independent of the clinician's perspectives*. While the clinician maintains the duty to educate the client on possibly phonotraumatic aspects of the client's preferred vocal approaches, the clinician must minimize judgment and bias regarding the client's choices. To this end, informed consent and the unbiased provision of information regarding vocal technique or approach facilitate rapport and trust between clinician and client.

Case Studies

How do all of these considerations come together? Please review the brief case studies below to see some of the various possibilities for goals, challenges, strengths, and intervention considerations. Also consider how one might employ a TIC lens and client-led service.

Client 1*: WS self-identifies as a "butch" lesbian transgender woman and uses she/her pronouns. She reports she is frequently misgendered and coded as a cis gay man in her communities. She wants to maintain a more masculine demeanor but more forward resonance in line with stereotypically feminine voice configurations. She describes her vocal target as "mouthy," "Valley Girl-like", and "sassy." WS alongside SLP identified goals related to increasing prosodic variation (*i.e.*, upspeak, prolongations), adjusting lingual articulation to be more forward facing (and incorporating final glottal stops for final /t/) in addition to forward resonance targets.*

Client 2*: SF uses she/they pronouns and has experienced self-reported trauma in response to ABA (Applied Behavior Analysis) intervention as a child. As a result, she is now resistant to drill-based, structured intervention. They are an autistic nonbinary transfeminine client who describes their voice as "monotonous." She is a 16-year-old at home with parents and disclosed they are "out" and parents encouraged them to seek voice services. They want to maintain forward resonance but she desires a lower pitch and "rougher" quality, but they feel self-conscious practicing at home.*

Client 3: *PJ is a Black, transfeminine client who uses she/her pronouns, and her work involves hauling large appliances to people's homes. She has been successful with modifying her habitual resonance and pitch in conversation but desires to modify these targets to address unsatisfied customers in her workplace to sound more "authoritative." She finds her previous habitual voice is manifested and worries about being misgendered. PJ's additional self-reported challenge in these situations is that she feels frustrated and emotional, making it difficult to use voice techniques in triggering moments.*

Client 4: *CK, a Korean-American transgender woman using she/her pronouns, is a self-described "perfectionist" who is employed as a data engineer. CK reports she is frequently cis-assumed but continues to feel uncomfortable with her voice despite progress and that frequency and resonance parameters appear in line with stereotypically cis feminine voice norms. SLP reinforces this feedback while recognizing the possible impact of gender dysphoria and makes recommendations for mental health counseling and transgender women's peer support groups, but CK is resistant. SLP elects to refer CK to a colleague for second opinion and further guidance.*

Common Issues when Interacting with TGNC Individuals

What happens if an employee in the clinician's institution misgenders their client? How can the relationship be repaired to assure the client that the space is safe and accountable? What should a clinician do if a client reports a negative experience in the waiting area? There are a number of solutions and approaches based on the client's comfort and general TGNC considerations for safety [15]. *Caveat: there is no uniform response to ameliorate or excuse the negative impact an employee can have on a TGNC individual due to lack of education, training, or knowledge.* Here are some common triggers and missteps and suggestions to manage them.

Misgendering or Deadnaming

Misgendering *is using incorrect pronouns or honorifics for an individual.*

Deadnaming *is using the name assigned at birth that the client no longer uses.*

If this done inadvertently, correct it quickly. Move on and model that the correct name and pronoun for the person are known. Do not apologize profusely or call undue attention to the situation – this prolongs the client's experience of feeling othered and triggered.

Triggering Topics

Focus on discussions that facilitate comfort and rapport in the clinical relationship and avoid triggering topics. Examples of triggering topics include, but are not limited to, religion, lifestyle, politics, holiday plans, marriage, parents, children, comments about diet, remarks about appearance, sexuality, surgical history, and transition. Generally safe topics include, but are not limited to, weather, hobbies, books, television, movies, music, leisure, and pets.

Responding When Someone Is Triggered

If there is an accidental touch on a painful point for a client, do not dig or inquire further. Follow their lead and move forward. Ask them whether it is ok to proceed with questioning, discussion, examination, or consideration. An example of how to do this is, "I didn't realize your family wasn't in the picture, I'm sorry to have brought that topic into our clinical space. Take as much time as you need to recenter. Should I continue with the interview or would you like to move on to another topic or activity?" If the client wants to discuss their pain point, listen empathically and offer supportive comments (e.g., "That must be very difficult," "I'm sorry you're going through that"), and do not center on personal experiences when responding (e.g., "My brother doesn't talk to the family either").

Considerations for Note and Report Writing

Ask clients how to refer to them in writing. Write without pronouns when there are discrepancies in official documentation. Use initial of first name and full last name (e.g., J. Patel) unless a client's documentation is consistent. Always ask: it is never known who will receive the report and how that may impact client safety.

Receiving Negative Feedback

If a client reports a negative experience with the clinic or institution, follow up in writing. Do not call and expect the client to recount their trauma over the phone, and do not question them nor excuse members of the staff for their mistreatment. Instead, send them an email and ask for a description of the issue. Once there has been a follow-up on the institution's misstep, then email the client and enact restorative practices. This can include emailing the client that the person perpetrating a microaggression has been trained, and what protocol was used, confirmation that their information in the institutional record system is updated and that no employee will misgender them in the future. Offer the patient how they would like to follow up, if at all via phone, email, or in person for the next appointment.

Ideally…

You enter a crowded clinic waiting room and check in. You give the name you used when registering in the online portal. The front desk staff hands you some paperwork. You easily fill in the form because it explicitly states "name we should call you" and "pronouns" on the top line. There are no binary choices. The form states, "please hand your ID to the front desk staff for our records, do not worry if your name differs from what is on the form." The safe space flags include the names of staff who have been formally trained and the certification agency. Your clinician's name is listed. There are no triggering questions, and the bathroom keys are on the desk with no binary markers. From behind a cracked door, a clinician you've never met calls out your name, and you see her pronouns clearly displayed on her ID. You think to yourself: "I can tell my friends to come here, and that never happens." This…is a safe, inclusive, and accountable space. This is a culturally responsive practice.

References

1. Reay B. Trans America: A Counter-History (1st ed.) [E-book]. Cambridge: Polity; 2020. https://doi.org/10.1093/jsh/shaa063.
2. Kozan, AL, Hammond SC. The Singing Voice. In: Adler RK, Hirsch S, Pickering J, editors. Voice and communication therapy for the transgender/gender diverse client: a comprehensive clinical guide. 3rd ed. San Diego, CA: Plural Publishing, Inc.; 2019.
3. Sanchez NF, Sanchez JP, Danoff A. Health care utilization, barriers to care, and hormone usage among male-to-female transgender persons in New York City. Am J Public Health. 2009;99:713–9. https://doi.org/10.2105/AJPH.2007.132035.
4. Minnican C, O'Toole G. Exploring the incidence of culturally responsive communication in Australian healthcare: the first rapid review on this concept. BMC Health Serv Res. 2020;20(1):20. https://doi.org/10.1186/s12913-019-4859-6.
5. Houssayni S, Nilsen K. Transgender competent provider: identifying transgender health needs, health disparities, and health coverage. Kans J Med. 2018;11(1):1–18. PMID: 29844850; PMCID: PMC5834239
6. Hendricks ML, Testa RJ. A conceptual framework for clinical work with transgender and gender nonconforming clients: an adaptation of the minority stress model. Prof Psychol Res Pract. 2012;43(5):460–7. https://doi.org/10.1037/a0029597.
7. Meyer IH. Prejudice, social stress, and mental health in lesbian, gay, and bisexual populations: conceptual issues and research evidence. Psychol Bull. 2003;129(5):674–97. https://doi.org/10.1037/0033-2909.129.5.674.

8. Testa RJ, Habarth J, Peta J, Balsam K, Bockting W. Development of the gender minority stress and resilience measure. Psychol Sex Orientat Gend Divers. 2015;2(1):65–77. https://doi.org/10.1037/sgd0000081.
9. Chart by the Institute on Trauma and Trauma-Informed Care. 2015
10. Grant JM, Mottet LA, Tanis J, Harrison J, Herman JL, Keisling M. Injustice at every turn: a report of the National Transgender Discrimination Survey. Washington, DC: National Center for Transgender Equality and National Gay and Lesbian Task Force; 2018.
11. Safer JD, Coleman E, Feldman J, Garofalo R, Hembree W, Radix A, Sevelius J. Barriers to healthcare for transgender individuals. Curr Opin Endocrinol Diabetes Obes. 2016;23(2):168–71. https://doi.org/10.1097/MED.0000000000000227.
12. Fink AS, Prochazka AV, Henderson WG, Bartenfeld D, Nyirenda C, Webb A, Berger DH, Itani K, Whitehill T, Edwards J, Wilson M, Karsonovich C, Parmelee P. Enhancement of surgical informed consent by addition of repeat back: a multicenter, randomized controlled clinical trial. Ann Surg. 2010;252(1):27–36.
13. Hall DE, et al. Informed consent for clinical treatment. CMAJ. 2012;184(5):533–40. https://doi.org/10.1503/cmaj.112120.
14. American Speech-Language-Hearing Association. Code of Ethics. American Speech-Language-Hearing Association (ASHA). 2016. https://www.asha.org/code-of-ethics/.
15. Burnes TR, Dexter MM, Richmond K, Singh AA, Cherrington A. The experiences of transgender survivors of trauma who undergo social and medical transition. Traumatology. 2016;22(1):75–84. https://doi.org/10.1037/trm0000064.

Chapter 5
Patient-Reported Outcomes and Data Collection in Treatment-Seeking Transgender and Gender Nonconforming Individuals

Maurice E. Goodwin, Ruchi Kapila, and Ry Pilchman

Introduction

As delineated by the American Speech-Language-Hearing Association (2017), the role of the speech-language pathologists (SLPs) is to provide culturally responsive services employing evidence-based practice (EBP) and clinical expertise with consideration for client perspectives as reflected by the World Health Organization International Classification of Functioning, Disability, and Health (WHO ICF) model. In recent years, the intention to integrate this clinical model and standard in the provision of gender-affirming voice services within the SLP scope has increasingly become a focus. The ICF model provides a framework for intervention from assessment, intervention planning, evaluation of efficacy of intervention, interdisciplinary communication between care providers, and, most importantly for this population, the self-evaluation of outcomes per the client or patient [1]. A caveat: unless

M. E. Goodwin (✉)
Houston Methodist's Department of Otolaryngology—Head and Neck Surgery, Houston Methodist Hospital, Houston, TX, USA
e-mail: mgoodwin@houstonmethodist.org

R. Kapila
Kapila Voice and Speech Services, Hayward, CA, USA

R. Pilchman
Rutgers University, Newark, NJ, USA

Robert Wood Johnson Barnabas Health, New Brunswick, NJ, USA

Prismatic Speech Services, New York, NY, USA
e-mail: ry.pilchman@rutgers.edu

M. S. Courey et al. (eds.), *Voice and Communication in Transgender and Gender Diverse Individuals*, https://doi.org/10.1007/978-3-031-24632-6_5

vocal fold pathology or overall medical compromise impacting respiration, phonation, or resonation is present, the authors will not use "treatment" or "therapy" to describe gender-affirming voice services and modification in this chapter.

ASHA asserts speech-language pathologists may be highly skilled vocal function specialists and play an integral role in the evaluation and care of clients, especially in the domain of disordered or atypically functioning voice production [2]. In an attempt to standardize and guide care providers in supporting clients' voice and communication needs, World Professional Association for Transgender Health (WPATH) officially recognized SLPs as the primary practitioner in the area of voice and communication for transgender and gender nonconforming (TGNC) individuals in their seventh version of Standards of Care (SOC 7) [3]. Per this publication, SLPs conduct and guide the majority, if not the entirety, of assessment and intervention protocols, including the collection of results of instrumental evaluation, acoustic and aerodynamic data, and patient-reported outcome measures (PROMs).

It is critical for the SLP to recognize that not all TGNC individuals seek voice modification as a part of embodying gender affirmation. It is key for the SLP to validate the subjective experiences of the TGNC client but to avoid describing their vocal presentation as "disordered" or "suboptimal" in the absence of pathology or medical compromise. In order for the SLP to center the client's experiences and perspectives adequately for gender-affirming voice care, training and investment in developing cultural responsiveness and trauma-informed care within the TGNC community are necessary to cultivate a safe and accountable space (see chapter on cultural responsiveness in TGNC community). If this model requirement is not met and continually updated, the SLP does not meet ASHA's nor WPATH's standards for culturally responsive care.

While this chapter is dedicated to identifying and discussing considerations for assessment and data collection when working with TGNC individuals whose voice goals and interventions may be habilitative, other voice professionals, voice teachers and coaches who are also TGNC community members, originated these services in gender-affirming voice modification. As SLPs it is essential to identify client-driven goals in consent-based care and to not assume. However, it is not uncommon for SLPs to assume fundamental frequency and resonance configuration targets on assuming the client's desired gender expression outcome, which can cause irrevocable harm to the TGNC individual. Gender-affirming voice work is an extremely personal endeavor that does not explicitly require the expertise of clinicians specializing in pathological or atypical voicing. Thus, this chapter will provide established data regarding gender perception and voice characteristics while prioritizing the perspectives of TGNC individuals seeking voice services, through the use of patient-reported outcome measures (PROMs) and other voice-related outcome data per the framework of the client, as markers of progress in gender-affirming voice modification.

What Are Patient-Reported Outcomes?

Measuring data throughout the diagnostic and treatment process plays an important role in adhering to current EBP and ICF models of care. In the area of voice training for TGNC individuals, data related to acoustic, aerodynamic, and auditory-perceptual measures take prominence throughout the literature. The prominence of these data often comes at the cost of the perspective of the individual or patient for whom the data represents. Many TGNC individuals seek voice training from speech pathologists for desired outcomes that may be unobservable as described by Cohen and Hula [4]. These unobservable outcomes may include perspectives such as effort, emotional discomfort, and patient confidence. While the previously mentioned objective data help demonstrate success as often measured by the clinician or treating SLP, the patient's own perspective of their health and treatment outcomes exists at the core of the ICF models of care. Patient-reported outcome measures (PROMs) are currently the most accurate and systematic way of measuring progress per the client's subjective experience [4].

Within the context of TGNC voice training in the traditional voice center model, it is important to emphasize a crucial issue in this model of care. Providers utilize data to demonstrate efficacy of provided therapeutic interventions. However, TGNC individuals have not historically relied on clinician-provided PROMs to measure their own progress and success with voice modification. In determining the role of objective data and PROMs within the framework of gender-affirming voice modification, it should be noted that these outcome measures were largely developed outside of the TGNC community.

Data Collection

In the traditional voice care model, any individual seeking intervention for concerns regarding their voice quality or function would participate in a comprehensive assessment, often including a series of standardized and non-standardized measures [5]. These measures, in compliance with the ICF framework, seek to measure any deficits, limitations, barriers, and impacts to quality of life for the individual presenting with a voice disorder. A cornerstone of the traditional voice evaluation includes outcome data, which this chapter seeks to delineate.

The use of acoustic, aerodynamic, auditory-perceptual, and patient-reported outcome measures in the context of voice evaluation will be deconstructed for the applicability to TGNC individuals, including analysis of data most documented within the current literature regarding voice intervention for this population.

Clinician-Perceived Dysphonia

In a retrospective chart review of 25 treatment-seeking transgender women at various stages of the transition, age, and educational level, Hancock and Garabedian [6] found that a perceived and measurable voice disorder was present in 28% of cases [6]. While this is a limited sample size and could not possibly represent all TGNC individuals, it does demonstrate the realities and prevalence of voice disorders in the general public. The prevalence of a voice problem or disorder at any point in an adult's life has been measured as high as 29.9% of a random sampling of adults of various genders between the age of 20 and 66 [7]. This data appears to be impacted by the gender, age, and occupation of the individual with the identified voice disorder [8]. As TGNC individuals are a part of the general population, it is expected that a provider may likely encounter an individual seeking voice modification services who presents with a clinician-perceived dysphonia.

Any provider concerned about the presence of dysphonia or perceived voice dysfunction should conduct an assessment based on relevant factors in the patient history and physical examination in conjunction with examination by an ear, nose, and throat (ENT) physician or laryngologist [9]. As established previously, the traditional and recommended evaluation for perceived dysphonia consists of various instrumental and non-instrumental assessments. Currently, there is no standardized formal voice assessment protocol adopted across all voice care providers. Barriers to standardization in voice evaluation include varied accessibility to trained providers with specialized equipment and different subspecialties and patient populations seen by voice care providers, necessitating adaptability in evaluation protocols. Recommended instrumental assessment of voice in the presence of dysphonia includes acoustic analysis, aerodynamic procedures, and laryngeal endoscopic imaging (Table 5.1, [10]). Non-instrumental assessment of voice often includes auditory-perceptual evaluation and patient self-assessment of voicing [5].

Table 5.1 Core tasks and measures for laryngeal imaging with valid regularity

Tasks	Light source	
	Continuous light	Strobe light
Rest breathing	Vocal fold edge	Vocal fold edge
• Three complete breath cycles (inhalation and exhalation)		
Laryngeal diadochokinetic task /?i?i?i?i?i/	Gross-level vocal fold mobility	Gross-level vocal fold mobility
Maximum-range vocal fold adduction and abduction during alternated /i:/-sniff or /i:/-quick inhale	Vocal fold mobility maximum range	Vocal fold mobility maximum range
Sustained phonation of /i:/ at stable typical pitch and loudness	Supraglottic compression	• Supraglottic compression
		• Regularity

Table 5.1 (continued)

Tasks	Light source	
	Continuous light	Strobe light
• At least three consecutive glottal cycles		• Amplitude
		• Mucosal wave
		• Left/right phase symmetry
		• Vertical level
		• Glottal closure pattern
		• Glottal closure duration
Sustained phonation of /i:/ at varied pitches (e.g., high, low pitch)	Supraglottic compression	• Supraglottic compression
		• Regularity
• At least three consecutive glottal cycles for each pitch variation		• Amplitude
		• Mucosal wave
		• Left/right phase symmetry
		• Vertical level
		• Glottal closure pattern
		• Glottal closure duration
Sustained phonation of /i:/ at varied loudness levels (e.g., loud voice, quiet voice production)	Supraglottic compression	• Supraglottic compression
		• Regularity
• At least three consecutive glottal cycles for each loudness variation		• Amplitude
		• Mucosal wave
		• Left/right phase symmetry
		• Vertical level
		• Glottal closure pattern
		• Glottal closure duration

Patel et al. Protocols for voice assessment

Normophonic Voicing

In the absence of dysphonia, outcome-related voice function and voice quality can be measured through acoustic, aerodynamic, auditory-perceptual, and patient self-reported tools. In the work of TGNC voice modification, the literature over-represents certain acoustic characteristics of voice such as fundamental frequency, which corresponds to the client's comfortable or desired speaking pitch. The first issue with over-prioritizing fundamental frequency is that many factors beyond pitch impact the perception of an individual's gender in their voice and overall presentation. Additionally, the standards for acoustic, aerodynamic, and auditory-perceptual evaluation related to gender have been largely pioneered and defined within a binary gender model (i.e., male or female), which does not adequately reflect the varied voice modification goals across the gender spectrum. Therefore, while acoustic measures may provide some information to the provider and patient, it is ultimately a patient's self-perception and assessment of voicing that is the gold standard for client-centered care.

Patient-Reported Outcome Measures (PROMs)

Patient-reported outcome measures (PROMs) are at the core of measuring success in the voice modification in TGNC individuals. As discussed, PROMs are the most accurate way of measuring the patient's perspective of their own voicing at all stages of care [4]. The literature is clear that self-perception of the voice for the TGNC person is an important measure to consider and has a large psychosocial impact on everyday life [11]. The Trans Woman Voice Questionnaire (TWVQ) (formally known as the Transsexual Voice Questionnaire or TVQ^{MtF}), Transgender Self-Evaluation Questionnaire (TSEQ), and Voice Handicap Index (VHI) have all been frequently documented as appropriate PROMs in measuring the TGNC perspective. Examples of these forms are available to review at the end of this chapter.

The Transgender Self-Evaluation Questionnaire (TSEQ) was developed and modeled after the Voice Handicap Index [12, 13]. The questionnaire consists of 30 statements where the individual completing the questionnaire rates their own experience on a 5-point Likert scale with 1 indicating "never" and 5 indicating "always." Statements include "My voice makes me feel less feminine (MtF) or masculine (FtM)" and "I feel my voice doesn't match my physical appearance." However, unlike the VHI, there is no categorization framework for rating severity of self-perceived voice limitations. A 2017 study conducted by Hancock demonstrated that the VHI and the TSEQ correlate fairly when aiming to measure self-perceived quality of life as defined by the ICF model of care [14]. The data also supported that the TSEQ may be more sensitive to the perceived limitations in transgender women and, therefore, serves as a more sensitive tool for measuring self-perceived voice-related quality of life.

The Trans Woman Voice Questionnaire (TWVQ) is a validated and reliable tool developed to specifically measure the voice-related quality of life (VRQOL) of transgender women [15]. Similar to the TSEQ, the questionnaire asks the individual to rate their self-perception across 30 statements on a 4-point Likert scale where a score of 1 equals "never or rarely" and a score of 4 equals "usually or always." Lower TWVQ scores indicated better voice-related quality of life. Researchers have tested the validity of the TWVQ in various populations of transgender women and found that the statement themes that emerge most prominently in the questionnaire correlated strongly with concerns expressed by these women [16–18]. Component analysis completed by Dacakis, Oates, and Douglas [17] revealed a two-factor structure to the TWVQ that could more accurately address areas of concern for transgender women based on their responses on the questionnaire. The first component, titled "voice functioning," contained 14 statements that demonstrated consistency with how participants perceived their voice function as well as items related to voice and gender identity. The second component, titled "social participation," consists of 12 of the items that related to the impact of voice on an individual's participation in activities of daily living [17]. By reviewing the TWVQ through this two-pronged lens, the authors were hopeful that goals and objectives related to voice function and presentation could be more accurately targeted based on responses provided.

Bultynck et al. [19] conducted a similar construct validity study and found the TWVQ demonstrated a three-component structure. Analysis was completed with 145 transgender women and 83 transgender men using an adapted version of the TWVQ for transgender men [20]. The three components were labeled as (1) anxiety and avoidance, (2) vocal identity, and (3) vocal function [19]. Similar to the study completed by Dacakis et al. [17], the goal in creating this three-component structure would be to more accurately measure self-perceived limitations and thus more accurately track improvement with intervention.

Finally, the Voice Handicap Index (VHI) and Voice Handicap Index-10 (VHI-10) are tools validated and developed to measure the impact of various voice disorders on an individual's quality of life [13, 21]. The VHI and VHI-10 are regularly used within the standard voice clinical model across all voice disorders. These questionnaires were not created nor validated on TGNC individuals; however Hancock [14] demonstrated fair correlation between TGNC-rated scores on the VHI and the TSEQ (A. B. [14]). A large survey study conducted by Kennedy and Thibeault [22] used the VHI as a tool for measuring the relationship between VHI scores and voice-gender incongruence across a spectrum of gender identity [22]. Across genders, voice-gender incongruence was significantly correlated with greater VHI scores indicating a greater self-perceived impact on QOL. This data further demonstrates the need for patient-specific outcome measures that aim to quantify the impact on voice-related quality of life. The VHI-10, a shortened ten-question version of the original VHI, has shown efficacy in measuring change post-operatively in the surgical management of voice modification [21, 23, 24].

PROMs can serve as a tool for measuring general feelings and attitudes that correlate with VRQOL. While these tools help us quantify the individual's feelings, as Hancock [14] asserted, "...participants can only answer the items provided on the questionnaire...it is possible that important questions are not included or asked" [14]. The role of a structured interview, alongside the implementation of PROMs, helps reveal the multifaceted and nuanced goals for the individual seeking voice modification.

Acoustic, Aerodynamic, and Auditory-Perceptual Evaluation

While much of the data regarding voice modification have placed a significant emphasis on the individual's speaking fundamental frequency, voice and communication is a multilayered and complex endeavor which frequently requires more than modification of pitch to produce a voice congruent with an individual's gender. Resonance, intonation, inflection, articulation, rate of speech, voice quality, and even airflow may all be features to address and consider in helping the individual achieve their optimal voice configuration. Collecting acoustic, aerodynamic, and auditory-perceptual data for these characteristics at baseline helps the clinician and the individual establish appropriate goals for voice modification.

Acoustic characteristics of voicing at baseline may include (1) fundamental frequency (f0), an individual's comfortable speaking pitch, (2) physiologic voice range (the maximum and minimum frequency achievable), (3) voice sound pressure level (SPL) across various stimuli (the measure of voice intensity in dB), (4) voice frequency standard deviation (a measure of voice intonation during speaking voice tasks), and (5) other quantitative voice quality measures such as cepstral peak prominence (CPP) and cepstral-spectral index of dysphonia (CSID). Aerodynamic measures of voicing include average glottal airflow rate and glottal air pressure for voicing in relationship with measures of SPL and frequency during the tasks (Table 5.2, [10]).

The clinician can use the Consensus Auditory-Perceptual Evaluation of Voice (CAPE-V) and the grade, roughness, breathiness, asthenia, and strain (GRBAS) rating scale as tools for evaluating the perceptual characteristics of a patient's voice quality. CAPE-V is a tool for clinicians to describe auditory-perceptual attributes of

Table 5.2 Core tasks and measures for acoustics analysis

Tasks	Acoustic measures
Sustained vowel for 3- to 5-s duration	• Cepstral peak prominence (CPP_{vowel})
• /a:/	
Standard reading passage	• Mean vocal frequency (Hz)
• Rainbow Passage (adults)	• Habitual vocal SPL (dB)
• "The Trip to the Zoo" passage (children)	• Vocal frequency standard deviation (Hz)
	• Cepstral peak prominence (CPP_{speech})
Loudness range	• Maximum vocal SPL (dB)
• Loudness glide on the vowel /a/, sustaining the loudest and quietest sounds for 1 s	• Minimum vocal SPL (dB)
Pitch range	• Maximum vocal frequency (Hz)
• Pitch glide on the vowel /a/, sustaining the highest and lowest pitches for 1 s	• Minimum vocal frequency (Hz)

Extracted from Patel et al. [10]

voice and levels of severity of any voice problems. It aids in hypothesizing whether further evaluation for potential vocal pathologies is warranted. The CAPE-V indicates salient perceptual vocal attributes such as (a) overall severity, (b) roughness, (c) breathiness, (d) strain, (e) pitch, and (f) loudness. The CAPE-V describes each attribute as mildly deviant, moderately deviant, and severely deviant. Ratings are based on the clinician's direct observations of the patient's performance during the evaluation, rather than patient report or other sources. The client completes three tasks: (1) sustaining vowel sounds /a/ and /i/ three times for 3–5 s, (2) reading six sentences designed to elicit various laryngeal behaviors (easy onset, hard glottal attacks, voiced, voiceless plosive sounds, and nasal sounds) and clinical signs, and (3) the client will produce 20 s of natural conversational speech using standard interview questions such as "tell me about your voice problem" [25]. The GRBAS (grade, roughness, breathiness, asthenia, and strain) uses a 4-point voice quality rating scale where "0" indicates normal, "1" mildly deviant, "2" moderately deviant, and "3" extremely deviant when the listener is observing a client producing sustained various vowel sounds and standardized reading passages (i.e., "The Rainbow Passage"). GRBAS is not a standardized measure of auditory perception, and CAPE-V is more frequently used [26].

Limitations in Determining Gender-Affirming Voice Targets from Cisgender Voice Norms (as Described in Table 5.3)

Many speech-language pathologists providing gender-affirming voice services use cisgender voice norms (e.g., speaking fundamental frequency (SFF), resonance configurations, prosodic characteristics, etc.) as described in current literature to

Table 5.3 Limitations in cisgender voice descriptions across studies

	Cisgender women	Cisgender men
Speaking fundamental frequency (SFF)	180–220hz[a] [3]	100–120hz[a] [3]
Resonance (F1/F2/F3)	All formants higher, based on shorter vocal tract length [27–29]	All formants lower, based on greater vocal tract length [27]
Intonation/inflection	Upward intonation [30, 31]	Flatter speech intonation [32]
Voice quality	Increased "breathiness" [12, 31]	Inconclusive
Articulation	Precise articulation [33, 34]	Greater imprecision in articulatory approximation [35]
Intensity	Reduced intensity [36, 37]	Average greater intensity than women [38]
Rate and prosody	Inconclusive	Inconclusive
Characteristics of airflow	Longer open phases [39, 40]	Higher amplitude-based flow parameters [39, 40]

[a]These values vary widely across numerous studies and ages of participants, as discussed in Adler et al. [41]

determine the course of voice intervention and assessment of efficacy of modification services. This table is included to elucidate the limitations in cisgender voice norm descriptions and current research. It is not necessary and may not be appropriate to include these measures in goal writing when working with the transgender and gender nonconforming (TGNC) community.

Using Acoustic/Aerodynamic/Perceptual Analysis for Pre- and Post-Operative Gender-Affirming Voice Surgery

PROMs and other points of data play an important role in measuring success for individuals seeking laryngeal surgery to permanently shift (i.e., raise) the pitch of their voice. Any procedure that changes the positioning, mass, or length of the vocal folds within the laryngeal mechanism has the ability to change the vibratory characteristics, thus having a greater impact to the pitch and related qualities of voicing. Similar to other laryngeal procedures, permanent changes to the larynx require significant preoperative and post-operative measurement of voice quality and function to determine patient- and clinician-perceived success. Without accurate pre-treatment baseline data, it would be difficult to justify surgical intervention and objectively measure success following such intervention, especially if changing fundamental frequency is the patient's primary focus.

It is also important to understand that post-operative complications in voice quality and function and not unheard of. Common post-operative complaints in individuals undergoing these procedures can include weakness in voice intensity, reduced vocal range, limited or abnormally elevated change in pitch, generalized dysphonia as measured on GRBAS scale, and increase in instability of voicing [42, 43].

One study measuring the impact of Wendler glottoplasty on vocal quality as measured across various frequently used acoustic measures (e.g., cepstral peak prominence [CPP], cepstral spectral index of dysphonia [CSID], and noise-to-harmonic ratio [NHR]) demonstrated stability in these measures post-operatively, indicating minimal change in voice quality per these acoustic measures regardless of perceived success in dramatically increasing the fundamental frequency [24]. Positively, within this same study population, analysis of PROMs (e.g., VHI-10, TWVQ) demonstrated statistically and clinically significant reduction in score, indicating patient-perceived improvement in function and presentation of voice. It should be noted that concomitant voice therapy throughout the voice transition process results in higher rates of patient-perceived satisfaction as well as elevated success for increased fundamental frequency [23, 44].

Regardless of objective measures of success in maintaining voice quality, it is important to prioritize patient-reported satisfaction with any treatment intervention in this population. Voice care teams must prioritize the functional outcomes for surgical patients as their ability to participate in activities of daily living (ADLs) with self-satisfaction in voicing holds the highest rating of success [45].

Conclusion

A comprehensive voice evaluation including acoustic and aerodynamic measures, videostroboscopic examination, and interview with measurement of patient- or client-reported outcomes is standard in developing an intervention plan for individuals with dysphonia. However, when TGNC individuals seek voice modification services for gender affirmation without a concern for vocal fold pathology, or overall medical compromise, voice care providers must critically assess and prioritize aspects of the voice evaluation in order to ensure client-centered goal formulation and service provision.

Per ASHA, and most interdisciplinary care standards, evidence-based practice supported by objective outcome data is key to ensure the efficacy of therapeutic or habilitative interventions. Yet, if objective outcome measures are utilized as a primary focus for intervention efficacy (as opposed to PROMs) when working with TGNC individuals on gender-affirming voice goals, it may negate the client's agency in determining optimal voice outcomes for themselves. It is recognized that ensuring insurance coverage for gender-affirming voice services, in addition to qualifying an individual for gender-affirming voice surgery, requires initial objective data collection to support an intervention. A greater emphasis may need to be placed on outcomes of PROMs in the future, to qualify an individual for service and procedure coverage, as well as describe the efficacy of an intervention modality.

Appendix

TWVQ

Rating Scale
1 = never or rarely
2 = sometimes
3 = often
4 = usually or always

Name: ____________________

Date: ____________________

Based on your actual experience of living as a female, please tick the response that fits you best.

		1	2	3	4
1.	People have difficulty hearing me in a noisy room.	☐	☐	☐	☐
2.	I feel anxious when I know I have to use my voice.	☐	☐	☐	☐
3.	My voice makes me feel less feminine than I would like.	☐	☐	☐	☐
4.	The pitch of my speaking voice is too low.	☐	☐	☐	☐
5.	The pitch of my voice is unreliable.	☐	☐	☐	☐
6.	My voice gets in the way of me living as a woman.	☐	☐	☐	☐
7.	I avoid using the phone because of my voice.	☐	☐	☐	☐
8.	I'm tense when talking with others because of my voice.	☐	☐	☐	☐
9.	My voice gets croaky, hoarse or husky when I try to speak in a female voice.	☐	☐	☐	☐
10.	My voice makes it hard for me to be identified as a woman.	☐	☐	☐	☐
11.	When I speak the pitch of my voice does not vary enough.	☐	☐	☐	☐
12.	I feel uncomfortable talking to friends, neighbours and relatives because of my voice.	☐	☐	☐	☐
13.	I avoid speaking in public because of my voice.	☐	☐	☐	☐
14.	My voice sounds artificial.	☐	☐	☐	☐
15.	I have to concentrate to make my voice sound the way I want it to sound.	☐	☐	☐	☐
16.	I feel frustrated with trying to change my voice.	☐	☐	☐	☐
17.	My voice difficulties restrict my social life.	☐	☐	☐	☐
18.	When I am not paying attention my pitch goes down.	☐	☐	☐	☐
19.	When I laugh I sound like a man.	☐	☐	☐	☐
20.	My voice doesn't match my physical appearance.	☐	☐	☐	☐
21.	I use a great deal of effort to produce my voice.	☐	☐	☐	☐
22.	My voice gets tired quickly.	☐	☐	☐	☐
23.	My voice restricts the sort of work I do.	☐	☐	☐	☐
24.	I feel my voice does not reflect the 'true me'.	☐	☐	☐	☐
25.	I am less outgoing because of my voice.	☐	☐	☐	☐
26.	I feel self-conscious about how strangers perceive my voice.	☐	☐	☐	☐
27.	My voice 'gives out' in the middle of speaking.	☐	☐	☐	☐
28.	It distresses me when I'm perceived as a man because of my voice.	☐	☐	☐	☐
29.	The pitch range of my speaking voice is restricted.	☐	☐	☐	☐
30.	I feel discriminated against because of my voice.	☐	☐	☐	☐

Please provide an overall rating of your voice:

Currently, my voice is:	☐ Very female	☐ Somewhat female	☐ Gender neutral	☐ Somewhat male	☐ Very male
My ideal voice would sound:	☐ Very female	☐ Somewhat female	☐ Gender neutral	☐ Somewhat male	☐ Very male

VOICE HANDICAP INDEX

Name:________________________ Date:________________

These are statements that many people have used to describe their voices and the effects of their voices on their lives. Circle the response that indicates how frequently you have the same experience.

0-never 1-almost never 2-sometimes 3-almost always 4-always

Part I-F

My voice makes it difficult for people to hear me.	0	1	2	3	4
People have difficulty understanding me in a noisy room.	0	1	2	3	4
My family has difficulty hearing me when I call them throughout the house.	0	1	2	3	4
I use the phone less often than I would like to.	0	1	2	3	4
I tend to avoid groups of people because of my voice.	0	1	2	3	4
I speak with friends, neighbors, or relatives less often because of my voice.	0	1	2	3	4
People ask me to repeat myself when speaking face-to-face.	0	1	2	3	4
My voice difficulties restrict my personal and social life.	0	1	2	3	4
I feel left out of conversations because of my voice.	0	1	2	3	4
My voice problem causes me to lose income.	0	1	2	3	4

1. SUBTOTAL _____

Part II-P

I run out of air when I talk.	0	1	2	3	4
The sound of my voice varies throughout the day.	0	1	2	3	4
People ask, "What's wrong with your voice?"	0	1	2	3	4
My voice sounds creaky and dry.	0	1	2	3	4
I feel as though I have to strain to produce voice.	0	1	2	3	4
The clarity of my voice is unpredictable.	0	1	2	3	4
I try to change my voice to sound different.	0	1	2	3	4
I use a great deal of effort to speak.	0	1	2	3	4
My voice is worse in the evening.	0	1	2	3	4
My voice "gives out" on me in the middle of speaking.	0	1	2	3	4

2. SUBTOTAL _____

Part III-E

	0	1	2	3	4
I am tense when talking to others because of my voice.	0	1	2	3	4
People seem irritated with my voice.	0	1	2	3	4
I find other people don't understand my voice problem.	0	1	2	3	4
My voice problem upsets me.	0	1	2	3	4
I am less outgoing because of my voice problem.	0	1	2	3	4
My voice makes me feels handicapped.	0	1	2	3	4
I feel annoyed when people ask me to repeat.	0	1	2	3	4
I feel embarrassed when people ask me to repeat.	0	1	2	3	4
My voice makes me feel incompetent.	0	1	2	3	4
I am ashamed of my voice problem.	0	1	2	3	4

3. SUBTOTAL ____

TOTAL__________

Score Range	Severity	Common Association
0-30	Mild	Minimal amount of handicap
31-60	Moderate	Often seen in patients with vocal nodules, polyps, or cysts
60-120	Severe	Often seen in patients with vocal fold paralysis or severe vocal fold scarring.

The Voice Handicap Index (VHI): Development and Validation. Barbara H. Jacobson, Alex Johnson, Cynthia Grywalski, Alice Silbergleit, Gary Jaconsen, Michael S. Benninger. American Journal of Speech-Language Pathology, Vol 6(3), 66-70, 1997, The Voice Handicap Index is reprinted with permission from all authors and ASHA.

Voice Handicap Index (VHI-10)

Name:________________________ Date:____________

Instructions: These are statements that many people have used to describe their voices and effects of their voices on their lives. Circle the response that indicates how frequently you have the same experience.

0 = never 1 = almost never 2 = sometimes 3 = almost always 4 = always

1. My voice makes it difficult for people to hear me.	0	1	2	3	4
2. I run out of air when I talk.	0	1	2	3	4
3. People have difficulty understanding me in a noisy room.	0	1	2	3	4
4. The sound of my voice varies throughout the day.	0	1	2	3	4
5. My family has difficulty hearing me when I call them throughout the house.	0	1	2	3	4
6. I use the phone less often than I would like to.	0	1	2	3	4
7. I'mtense when talking to others because of my voice.	0	1	2	3	4
8. I tend to avoid groups of people because of my voice.	0	1	2	3	4
9. People seem irritated with my voice.	0	1	2	3	4
10. People ask, "What's wrong with your voice?"	0	1	2	3	4

Rosen, C, Lee, A, Osborne, J, Zullo, T, and Murry, T (2004). Development and Validation of the Voice Handicap Index-10. Laryngoscope: 114(9): 1549-1556

Transgender Self Evaluation Questionnaire

How do you rate your voice? (overall)

Currently my voice is:	My ideal voice would sound:
O Very female	O Very female
O Somewhat female	O Somewhat female
O Gender neutral	O Gender neutral
O Somewhat male	O Somewhat male
O Very male	O Very male

RATING SCALE

1 = never
2 = almost never
3 = sometimes
4 = almost always
5 = always

How often do you experience the following?

				1	2	3	4	5	
F	1	People have difficulty hearing me in a noisy room.	never	O	O	O	O	O	always
P	2	I have trouble finding a vocal range that feels authentic to me.	never	O	O	O	O	O	always
E	3	My voice makes me feel less feminine(MTF)/masculine(FTM).	never	O	O	O	O	O	always
F	4	I feel the pitch range of my voice is restricted.	never	O	O	O	O	O	always
P	5	The sound of my voice varies throughout the day.	never	O	O	O	O	O	always
F	6	I feel my voice gets in the way of me living as a woman(ry1TF)/man(FTM).	never	O	O	O	O	O	always
F	7	I use the phone less often than I would like.	never	O	O	O	O	O	always
E	8	I'm tense when talking with others because of my voice.	never	O	O	O	O	O	always
E	9	I tend to avoid groups of people because of my voice.	never	O	O	O	O	O	always
E	10	People seem irritated with my voice.	never	O	O	O	O	O	always
P	11	People ask, "What's wrong with your voice?"	never	O	O	O	O	O	always
F	12	I speak with friends, neighbours and relatives less often because of my voice.	never	O	O	O	O	O	always
F	13	I avoid speaking in public because of my voice.	never	O	O	O	O	O	always
P	14	I feel my voice sounds artificial to others.	never	O	O	O	O	O	always
P	15	I have to strain to make my voice sound like I want it to.	never	O	O	O	O	O	always
E	16	I feel frustrated with trying to change my voice.	never	O	O	O	O	O	always
F	17	My voice difficulties restrict my personal and social life.	never	O	O	O	O	O	always
P	18	The pitch of my voice is unreliable_	never	O	O	O	O	O	always
P	19	When I laugh, cough or sneeze, I sound like a man(MTF)/ woman(FTM).	never	O	O	O	O	O	always
F	20	I feel my voice doesn't match my physical appearance.	never	O	O	O	O	O	always
P	21	I use a great deal of effort to speak.	never	O	O	O	O	O	always
P	22	My voice is worse in the evening.	never	O	O	O	O	O	always
F	23	My voice causes me to lose income.	never	O	O	O	O	O	always
E	24	I don't feel my voice reflects the "true me".	never	O	O	O	O	O	always
E	25	I am less outgoing because of my voice.	never	O	O	O	O	O	always
E	26	I feel self-conscious about how strangers perceive my voice.	never	O	O	O	O	O	always
P	27	My voice -gives out" in the middle of speaking.	never	O	O	O	O	O	always
E	28	I find it upsetting when I'm perceived as a man(MTF)/ woman(FTM) on the phone.	never	O	O	O	O	O	always
E	29	I am envious of other women(MTF)/men(FTM) who have more feminine(MTF)Imasculine(FTM) voices than mine.	never	O	O	O	O	O	always
E	30	My voice embarrasses me.	never	O	O	O	O	O	always

Shelagh Davies, 2012

References

1. World Health Organization. International classification of functioning, disability and health: ICF (p. Title of Beta 2, full version: international class). World Health Organization; 2001.
2. Association AS-L-H. Voice disorders. Practice Portal. n.d.

3. Davies S, Papp VG, Antoni C. Voice and communication change for gender nonconforming individuals: giving voice to the person inside. Int J Transgend. 2015;16(3) https://doi.org/10.1080/15532739.2015.1075931.
4. Cohen ML, Hula WD. Patient-reported outcomes and evidence-based practice in speech-language pathology. Am J Speech Lang Pathol. 2020;29(1) https://doi.org/10.1044/2019_AJSLP-19-00076.
5. Roy N, Barkmeier-Kraemer J, Eadie T, Sivasankar MP, Mehta D, Paul D, Hillman R. Evidence-based clinical voice assessment: A systematic review. Am J Speech Lang Pathol. 2013;22(2) https://doi.org/10.1044/1058-0360(2012/12-0014).
6. Hancock AB, Garabedian LM. Transgender voice and communication treatment: a retrospective chart review of 25 cases. Int J Lang Commun Disord. 2013;48(1) https://doi.org/10.1111/j.1460-6984.2012.00185.x.
7. Roy N, Merrill RM, Gray SD, Smith EM. Voice disorders in the general population: prevalence, risk factors, and occupational impact. Laryngoscope. 2005;115(11) https://doi.org/10.1097/01.mlg.0000179174.32345.41.
8. Cohen SM, Kim J, Roy N, Asche C, Courey M. Prevalence and causes of dysphonia in a large treatment-seeking population. Laryngoscope. 2012;122(2) https://doi.org/10.1002/lary.22426.
9. Stachler RJ, Francis DO, Schwartz SR, Damask CC, Digoy GP, Krouse HJ, McCoy SJ, Ouellette DR, Patel RR, Reavis CW, Smith LJ, Smith M, Strode SW, Woo P, Nnacheta LC. Clinical practice guideline: hoarseness (dysphonia) (update). Otolaryngol Head Neck Surg. 2018;158(1_suppl) https://doi.org/10.1177/0194599817751030.
10. Patel RR, Awan SN, Barkmeier-Kraemer J, Courey M, Deliyski D, Eadie T, Paul D, Švec JG, Hillman R. Recommended protocols for instrumental assessment of voice: American speech-language-hearing association expert panel to develop a protocol for instrumental assessment of vocal function. Am J Speech Lang Pathol. 2018;27(3) https://doi.org/10.1044/2018_AJSLP-17-0009.
11. Bultynck C, Pas C, Defreyne J, Cosyns M, den Heijer M, T'Sjoen G. Self-perception of voice in transgender persons during cross-sex hormone therapy. Laryngoscope. 2017;127(12) https://doi.org/10.1002/lary.26716.
12. Davies S, Goldberg JM. Clinical aspects of transgender speech feminization and masculinization. Int J Transgend. 2006;9(3–4) https://doi.org/10.1300/J485v09n03_08.
13. Jacobson BH, Johnson A, Grywalski C, Silbergleit A, Jacobson G, Benninger MS, Newman CW. The voice handicap index (VHI). Am J Speech Lang Pathol. 1997;6(3) https://doi.org/10.1044/1058-0360.0603.66.
14. Hancock AB. An ICF perspective on voice-related quality of life of American transgender women. J Voice. 2017;31(1) https://doi.org/10.1016/j.jvoice.2016.03.013.
15. Dacakis G, Davies S, Oates JM, Douglas JM, Johnston JR. Development and preliminary evaluation of the transsexual voice questionnaire for male-to-female transsexuals. J Voice. 2013;27(3) https://doi.org/10.1016/j.jvoice.2012.11.005.
16. Dacakis G, Oates JM, Douglas JM. Exploring the validity of the transsexual voice questionnaire (male-to-female): do TVQ MtF scores differentiate between MtF women who have had gender reassignment surgery and those who have not? Int J Transgend. 2016;17(3–4) https://doi.org/10.1080/15532739.2016.1222922.
17. Dacakis G, Oates JM, Douglas JM. Further evidence of the construct validity of the transsexual voice questionnaire (TVQ MtF) using principal components analysis. J Voice. 2017;31(2) https://doi.org/10.1016/j.jvoice.2016.07.001.
18. Davies SM, Johnston JR. Exploring the validity of the transsexual voice questionnaire for male-to-female transsexuals. Can J Speech Lang Pathol Audiol. 2015;39(1):40–51.
19. Bultynck C, Pas C, Defreyne J, Cosyns M, T'Sjoen G. Organizing the voice questionnaire for transgender persons. Int J Transgender Health. 2020;21(1) https://doi.org/10.1080/15532739.2019.1605555.
20. Kreukels BPC, Haraldsen IR, De Cuypere G, Richter-Appelt H, Gijs L, Cohen-Kettenis PT. A European network for the investigation of gender incongruence: the ENIGI initiative. Eur Psychiatry. 2012;27(6) https://doi.org/10.1016/j.eurpsy.2010.04.009.

21. Rosen CA, Lee AS, Osborne J, Zullo T, Murry T. Development and validation of the voice handicap Index-10. Laryngoscope. 2004;114(9) https://doi.org/10.1097/00005537-200409000-00009.
22. Kennedy E, Thibeault SL. Voice–gender incongruence and voice health information–seeking behaviors in the transgender community. Am J Speech Lang Pathol. 2020;29(3) https://doi.org/10.1044/2020_AJSLP-19-00188.
23. Brown SK, Chang J, Hu S, Sivakumar G, Sataluri M, Goldberg L, Courey MS. Addition of Wendler glottoplasty to voice therapy improves trans female voice outcomes. Laryngoscope. 2020; https://doi.org/10.1002/lary.29050.
24. Chang J, Brown SK, Hu S, Sivakumar G, Sataluri M, Goldberg L, Courey MS. Effect of Wendler glottoplasty on acoustic measures of voice. Laryngoscope. 2021;131(3) https://doi.org/10.1002/lary.28764.
25. Kempster GB, Gerratt BR, Verdolini Abbott K, Barkmeier-Kraemer J, Hillman RE. Consensus auditory-perceptual evaluation of voice: development of a standardized clinical protocol. Am J Speech Lang Pathol. 2009;18(2) https://doi.org/10.1044/1058-0360(2008/08-0017).
26. Sapienza, C. M., & Hoffman-Ruddy, B.. Chapter 4: Evaluation. Voice disorders. Essay. Plural Publishing; 2018.
27. Hillenbrand JM, Clark MJ. The role of f 0 and formant frequencies in distinguishing the voices of men and women. Atten Percept Psychophys. 2009;71(5) https://doi.org/10.3758/APP.71.5.1150.
28. Gelfer MP, Bennett QE. Speaking fundamental frequency and vowel formant frequencies: effects on perception of gender. J Voice. 2013;27(5) https://doi.org/10.1016/j.jvoice.2012.11.008.
29. Gelfer MP, Mikos VA. The relative contributions of speaking fundamental frequency and formant frequencies to gender identification based on isolated vowels. J Voice. 2005;19(4) https://doi.org/10.1016/j.jvoice.2004.10.006.
30. Hancock A, Colton L, Douglas F. Intonation and gender perception: applications for transgender speakers. J Voice. 2014;28(2) https://doi.org/10.1016/j.jvoice.2013.08.009.
31. Owen K, Hancock AB. The role of self- and listener perceptions of femininity in voice therapy. Int J Transgend. 2010;12(4) https://doi.org/10.1080/15532739.2010.550767.
32. Pickering L, Hu G, Baker A. The pragmatic function of intonation: cueing agreement and disagreement in spoken English discourse and implications for ELT. In: Romero-Trillo J, editor. Pragmatics and prosody in English language teaching; 2012. p. 199–218. https://doi.org/10.1007/978-94-007-3883-6_12.
33. Dacakis G, Oates J, Douglas J. Beyond voice. Curr Opin Otolaryngol Head Neck Surg. 2012;20(3) https://doi.org/10.1097/MOO.0b013e3283530f85.
34. Oates JM, Dacakis G. Speech pathology considerations in the management of transsexualism–a review. Int J Lang Commun Disord. 1983;18(3) https://doi.org/10.3109/13682828309012237.
35. Kempe V, Puts DA, Cárdenas RA. Masculine men articulate less clearly. Hum Nat. 2013;24(4) https://doi.org/10.1007/s12110-013-9183-y.
36. Holmberg EB, Oates J, Dacakis G, Grant C. Phonetograms, aerodynamic measurements, self-evaluations, and auditory perceptual ratings of male-to-female transsexual voice. J Voice. 2010;24(5) https://doi.org/10.1016/j.jvoice.2009.02.002.
37. Boonin J. Articulation. In: Adler RK, Hirsch S, Mordaunt M, editors. Voice and communication therapy for the transgender/transsexual client: A comprehensive clinical guide. 2nd ed. San Diego, CA: Plural; 2012. p. 249–62.
38. Pausewang Gelfer M, Young SR. Comparisons of intensity measures and their stability in male and female sneakers. J Voice. 1997;11(2):178–86. https://doi.org/10.1016/s0892-1997(97)80076-8.
39. Justine V. Goozee, Bruce E. Murdoch, Deborah G. Theodoros, Elizabeth C. Thompson. (1998). Notes and discussion the effects of age and gender on laryngeal aerodynamics. Int J Lang Commun Disord, 33(2). doi: https://doi.org/10.1080/136828298247884.

40. Stathopoulos ET, Sapienza CM. Developmental changes in laryngeal and respiratory function with variations in sound pressure level. J Speech Lang Hear Res. 1997;40(3) https://doi.org/10.1044/jslhr.4003.595.
41. Adler RK, Hirsch S, Pickering J. Voice and communication therapy for the transgender/gender diverse client: a comprehensive clinical guide. Plural Publishing Inc.; 2019.
42. Aires MM, Marinho CB, Souza CDSC. Effect of endoscopic glottoplasty on acoustic measures and quality of voice: A systematic review and meta-analysis. J Voice. 2020; https://doi.org/10.1016/j.jvoice.2020.11.005.
43. Song TE, Jiang N. Transgender phonosurgery: A systematic review and meta-analysis. Otolaryngol Head Neck Surg. 2017;156(5) https://doi.org/10.1177/0194599817697050.
44. Nolan IT, Morrison SD, Arowojolu O, Crowe CS, Massie JP, Adler RK, Chaiet SR, Francis DO. The role of voice therapy and phonosurgery in transgender vocal feminization. J Craniofac Surg. 2019;30(5) https://doi.org/10.1097/SCS.0000000000005132.
45. Morrison SD, Crowe CS, Rashidi V, Massie JP, Chaiet SR, Francis DO. Beyond phonosurgery: considerations for patient-reported outcomes and speech therapy in transgender vocal feminization. Otolaryngol Head Neck Surg. 2017;157(2) https://doi.org/10.1177/0194599817712678.

Part II
Behavioral Interventions to Aid Transition

Chapter 6
Applying Flow Phonation in Voice Care for Transgender Women, Nonbinary, and Gender Nonconforming Individuals

Sarah L. Schneider

Introduction

Breath is the life force for our bodies and the power source for our voice. Breath is key in achieving efficient, flexible, and dynamic voice production. Variations in airflow during phonation play a role in altering vocal quality ranging from breathiness to vocal roughness to pressed phonation. Variations in airflow also play a role in dynamic changes in vocal intensity. Traditionally, therapies or voice techniques targeting airflow work to rebalance the three subsystems of voice production to achieve balanced phonatory airflow and oral/nasal resonance resulting in an efficient and sustainable voice. Techniques may be used for voice rehabilitation in the setting of vocal fold lesions, a vocal fold motion impairment, or muscle tension dysphonia. In the context of gender affirming voice care, these same voice techniques not only help rebalance the subsystems of voice production to achieve efficient voicing but can be used in a habilitative context to explore the voice and vocal variables that may be gender affirmative. Vocal variables include pitch, resonance, intensity, intonation, and vocal flexibility, to name a few. Regardless of gender, all voice is made on the exhalation, and through this chapter, we will explore the role airflow plays, in isolation and then coordinated with phonation, in achieving gender affirming voice and communication.

S. L. Schneider (✉)
Department of Otolaryngology Head and Neck Surgery, University of California San Francisco, San Francisco, CA, USA
e-mail: sarah.schneider@ucsf.edu

M. S. Courey et al. (eds.), *Voice and Communication in Transgender and Gender Diverse Individuals*, https://doi.org/10.1007/978-3-031-24632-6_6

Background

"Flow phonation" is sometimes used colloquially in the field of speech-language pathology (SLP) when referring to exercises that focus on airflow during voice production. The voice exercises or techniques covered in this chapter fall under the umbrella of "flow phonation" and include stretch and flow phonation or stretch and flow voice therapy (SnF), flow phonation (FP), and, possibly, semi-occluded vocal tract (SOVT) exercises. To understand these techniques, it is important to recognize that types of voicing are described to range from breathy to pressed phonation and include breathy, flow, neutral, and pressed. These types of phonation are identified by their glottal airflow as measured by glottal inverse filtering [1, 2]. In typical conversational speech, neutral phonation is used, and complete or near-complete vocal fold closure is achieved. Breathy phonation is produced without vocal fold closure, whereas pressed phonation is produced with complete vocal fold closure and increased muscular force and effort. Flow phonation, however, has higher airflow than neutral phonation but less than breathy phonation, and during flow phonation touch vocal fold closure is achieved [1, 2].

Pre-dating the instrumental assessment of flow phonation which aids in our understanding of vocal fold closure during various voice production types, Stone and Casteel [3] introduced stretch and flow phonation as a therapeutic technique to address hyperfunctional voice use patterns. This technique targets exhalation initially in isolation and then coordinated with phonation while maintaining minimal vocal effort. Originally, this technique was used for people with muscle tension aphonia/dysphonia, and over the years, it has been integrated into more common practice in voice therapy across diagnoses (e.g., benign vocal fold lesions, vocal fold motion impairment) and in gender affirming voice work. Watts and colleagues have done a series of studies using stretch and flow voice therapy (SnF) which is based on stretch and flow phonation (SnF will be used to represent both stretch and flow phonation and stretch and flow voice therapy throughout this chapter). They found that SnF is efficacious as a treatment technique for muscle tension dysphonia and phonotraumatic vocal fold lesions [4, 5]. Additionally, in a randomized control trial, SnF was found not to be inferior to resonant voice therapy (RVT), another common voice therapy technique focused on achieving increased oral resonance to optimize voice production [6]. This is a powerful finding as there is a wide variety of evidence supporting the efficacy and clinical utility of RVT.

Stretch and flow phonation (SnF) has also been referred to as flow phonation (FP). However, FP and SnF should not be used interchangeably as different glottal configurations are used during each technique [2]. Gartner-Schmidt [7] describes FP as a modification of stretch and flow phonation. Traditionally, in SnF a voiceless and voiced /u/ are used to establish an air-filled and easy voice in a hierarchical fashion. With FP, this is also the case; however many combinations of voiceless and voiced sounds can be used, then combined with articulation working toward "clear speech," and ultimately used for carryover into conversational speech [7]. During

SnF, initially a breathy voice production is used; however with FP airflow from a breathy voice production is maintained but without a breathy quality. This is in line with Gauffin and Sundberg's [1] description that complete glottic closure is achieved during flow phonation. When working on both SnF and FP, visual feedback with a tissue to monitor airflow or kinesthetic feedback feeling airflow with a finger can be quite useful. Additionally, negative practice can play a role in helping the client develop volitional control over variations in airflow. This is not only helpful from a biomechanical standpoint to achieve airflow and optimize vocal fold closure but also to encourage the development of agency and self-efficacy for the client.

Semi-occluded vocal tract (SOVT) exercises, which may include humming, fricatives (e.g., /v/, /z/), straw phonation, straw phonation in water, tongue-out trills, tongue trills, and lip trills, as described by Titze in 2006, could also be considered loosely under the umbrella of "flow phonation." SOVT can be used to target coordination of breathing and phonation and to achieve consistent exhalation of airflow during phonation. SOVT exercises are completed with some form of narrowing at the front of the mouth creating increased intraoral pressure (back pressure). With this back pressure, the vocal tract shape is altered, the shape of the vocal folds is squared off, and subglottic pressure at the onset of phonation is reduced. Altogether, this decreases the impact force of vocal fold vibration [8].

Titze et al. [9] assessed straw phonation with different straw diameters to determine the effects during phonation. It is proposed that lung pressure increases with smaller-diameter straws but larger amplitude of vocal fold vibration nor longer length of vocal fold closure during phonation was observed [9]. And subsequently, pressed phonation may not be possible during straw phonation [9]. Kapsner-Smith et al. [10], in a randomized control study, found that SOVT exercises with flow resistance tubes (FRT) (like straw phonation) were efficacious and not inferior to vocal function exercises (VFE), a well-established voice exercise program using SOVT postures.

SOVT exercises work to optimize source (phonation)-filter (vocal tract) interaction to maximize "vocal economy" [8, 11]. Through this work consistent airflow is required, and sensations of oral/nasal resonance are heightened with increased vibration in bones of the face. Titze [8] suggests vocal training may be most efficient moving from greatest semi-occlusion to least semi-occlusion (Fig. 6.1). Training, monitoring and maintaining the sensations of airflow, resonance, and back pressure allow one to move toward more functional application (e.g., applying to conversational speech). It should be noted that when initiating any therapeutic technique, the clinician should assess the client's voice use patterns and begin at a level that is most successful for them, whether this is more or less semi-occluded.

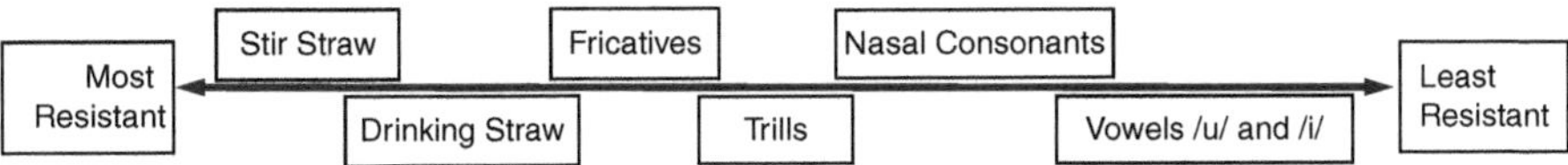

Fig. 6.1 Semi-occluded vocal tract exercises in order of intraoral resistance

Airflow Considerations with Transgender and Gender Nonconforming Individuals

Voice, regardless of gender, is achieved by activating and balancing the three subsystems of voice production including the power source (air from the lungs), sound source (vocal fold vibration), and the filter (how sound is amplified or damped by the shape of the vocal tract, called resonance). Variations in lung pressure, vocal fold vibration and closure, and resonance all impact how the voice sounds, is perceived by the individual voice user, and then is ultimately perceived by the listener. At the core of each of the airflow exercises, SnF, FP, and SOVT work to rebalance the three subsystems of voice production to optimize voice production whether for rehabilitation or habilitation.

When working to achieve congruence between voice, communication, and gender, understanding the interaction of the subsystems of voice production in relation to the anatomy and physiology and voice science is crucial. People present with different life experiences and various voice use patterns, and they may seek different outcomes related to their voice and communication. For example, increasing breathiness, lowering vocal intensity, and avoiding vocal fry are reported to contribute to a more feminine sounding voice [12–14]. Flow phonation could aid in altering these variables; however, it is key that they align with the client's goals. The journey through voice and communication therapy is a dynamic and multidimensional process. The focus of this chapter is related to airflow and patterns which can present on a spectrum from increased airflow (e.g., breathy voice), reduced airflow (e.g., vocal roughness or pressed phonation), or discoordination of breathing and phonation (e.g., which may result in a quality from breathy to pressed). Exploring the relationship between airflow and vocal quality, resonance, vocal intensity, vocal flexibility, and intonation patterns in the context of gender affirming voice care can help increase awareness of the role that variations in airflow play in voice production. When balanced airflow is not achieved, a person may have limited access to altering other vocal variables.

People can sometimes develop imbalanced phonatory airflow and muscle activation that leads to voice quality changes, vocal fatigue, discomfort, or even pain associated with voice use. It should be noted that frequent, prolonged, or habitual use of pressed phonation is thought to lead to a voice disorder due to a higher impact of vocal fold vibration [15]. Targeting airflow and coordination of breathing and phonation can help address inefficient voice use patterns while allowing for, or even promoting, changes in other vocal variables in a biomechanically efficient way.

Exploring Techniques to Facilitate Phonatory Airflow

Within each technique, SnF, FP, and SOVT, there are factors that may be more effective for one person than another based on individual voice use patterns, experience with their voice, previous voice training, and kinesthetic awareness, to name a few. It is important to be open to exploration and modifications within each technique. The clinician's understanding of the foundations of voice production, along with observing the client's voice use patterns can allow the clinician to work creatively within the voice techniques and help ensure the client connects with techniques that can be incorporated into everyday use.

SnF works through a hierarchy of exercises with increasing complexity up to conversational speech. It is initiated with breath in isolation and then coordinated with phonation on a /u/ vowel [3, 4]. As shown earlier (see Fig. 6.1), /u/ is a semi-occluded vowel with the least intraoral pressure compared to other SOVT exercises. Variations of SnF are not described in the literature. FP, however, is described by Gartner-Schmidt [7, 16] to have many variations that are initially completed in a voiceless fashion to establish airflow in isolation and then coordinated with phonation while maintaining necessary airflow. FP may incorporate /u/, gargling, trills (lip bubbles, tongue-out trills, tongue trills), and prolonged fricatives (/v/, /z/, /j/). The clinician works from airflow release to breathy phonation to flow phonation to articulatory precision and ultimately into conversational speech [7] guiding the client to find a balance that works for them.

SOVT exercises may also be achieved using more or less intraoral pressure (see Fig. 6.1). Variations include straw phonation with different diameter straws, cup bubbles (immersing a straw in water producing bubbles during exhalation and then phonation), Lax Vox (using a silicone tube in water) [17], trills, and voiced and voiceless fricatives (/f, v, s, z, ʃ, j/). SOVT exercises are often used at the phoneme level with less focus on carryover or application in conversational speech [8]. In clinical practice, the connection between voice exercise and "real-world" voice use is key to integrating new gender affirmative voice use patterns into daily life. SOVT exercises can be used as a facilitator into words, phrases, etc., just as SnF and FP connect the exercises to spoken words (see Table 6.1).

Table 6.1 Considerations from hierarchy to carryover

Technique	Facilitator	Establish airflow	Phoneme[a]	Words, phrases, sentences	Q&A/conversation
Stretch and flow phonation	/u/	Blow air on tissue or hand	Add voice on air-filled and easy /u/ vowel (airflow may vary from breathy to more balanced)	/u/ → /w/ words or words with initial vowels	/u/ → structured Q&A/ conversation; fade /u/ as able
Flow phonation	/u/	Blow air on tissue or hand	Add voice on /u, i, a/, move to articulation, e.g., poo-loo	/u/ → /w/ words or words with initial vowels	/u/ → structured Q&A/ conversation; fade /u/ as able
	Gargling	Voiceless gargle	Voiced gargle – explore speech like intonation Gradually tilt the head forward during the gargle letting water come into the mouth and make /m/ or swallow water and /a/	Gargle or /m/ or /a/ → words, etc.	Gargle or /m/ or /a/ → Q&A/ conversation; fade gargle as able
	Trills	Voiceless trill	Voiced trill	Trill → "br" words, etc. (e.g., bring, bring me some water)	Trill → structured Q&A or conversation; fade trill as able
	Fricatives	/f/, /s/, /ʃ/	Add voice on /v/, /z/, and /j/	Fricative → words, etc.	Fricative → as above; fade as able

SOVT	Straw phonation	Blow consistent air into the straw; explore the sensation of back pressure, achieve consistent airflow through straw	Add voice on an /u/ or /m/ into the straw; continue to explore sensation of back pressure, maintain consistent airflow through the straw, and find buzz at the Lips/straw	Straw talking → say a word, phrase, or sentence into the straw 3×, remove the straw, and say the same phrase while maintaining ease, quality, and pitch	Straw talking → as above; fade straw as able or alternately talk and use straw as needed to "*reset*"
	Cup bubbles	Blow consistent air into the straw in water; explore as above keeping consistent bubbles in the water	Add voice on an /u/ or /m/ into the straw in water; explore as above keeping consistent bubbles in the water	Straw talking → say a word, phrase, or sentence into the straw 3×, remove the straw from the water, do the same thing, remove the straw, and say the same phrase while maintaining ease, quality, and pitch	Straw talking → as above; fade cup bubbles/straw as able or alternately talk and use straw/cup bubbles as needed to "reset"
	Trills	Voiceless trill	Voiced trill	Lip trill → "br" words Tongue trill → "r" words Tongue-out trill → /m/ words	Fade use of trill as able or talk and use the trill as needed to "reset"
	Fricatives	As above with fricatives for flow phonation with increased focus on sensation of back pressure			
	/u/ or /i/	Voiceless blowing/exhalation	Voiced on /u/ or /i/ exploring sensation of back pressure/sound in the mouth	/u/ or /i/ → /w/ words or those that begin with vowels	/u/ or /i/ → Q&A and conversation; fade /u/ or /i/ as able or use as needed to "reset"

Reset—to return to the target voice by using a facilitator, taking a step back in the hierarchy, or bringing the attention back to the target to "reset"

[a]Using sustained sounds, glides, and sirens begin to explore pitch while maintaining airflow and ease. Identify a comfortable pitch range/target pitch range that aligns with the client's goals. For some, accessing a pitch in the "goal" range may be easily accessible right away, and for others it may be a step-wise process working up or down from the habitual speaking pitch. Work to explore and find the desired/comfortable pitch through the subsequent steps

From Structured Tasks to Generalization

Introducing airflow in isolation lays the foundation for the role the vocal folds play as a valve on top of the lungs [18] and can help increase awareness of breathing patterns (e.g., breath holding, tongue retraction, activation of neck muscles, etc.). While working on breathing in isolation, attention can be brought to the feelings in the throat. Is the throat open, narrow, tight, easy, etc.? Observing what may be happening in the jaw or the tongue can also be illuminating. Working to reduce overactivation in the throat, tongue, and jaw establishes a foundation to make voicing "as easy as breathing." In a complimentary fashion, focus can be brought to posture and body alignment, feeling the breath "in the body." The focus could be on thoracic and lower rib cage breathing, "abdominal" breathing, or reducing clavicular breathing that may contribute to tension patterns. Some clients wear body-shaping garments to alter the shape and appearance of their body and to address related dysphoria. These garments may in turn impact breathing [19]. It is important to be mindful when exploring breathing and allow the client space to express their comfort level with this work.

Once easy breathing is established, it is then coordinated with phonation. If there are pitch targets, they can be incorporated into work with all flow phonation techniques. Pairing flow phonation with pitch alteration helps connect these two components or variables as part of the whole, the whole in this case being voice production ultimately into conversational speech. Motor learning theory supports this idea of working on the whole or more complex tasks. While short-term trials may at times be more challenging, it is instrumental for long-term retention [20]. Below you will find an example of a hierarchy used to facilitate implementation of SnF incorporating pitch targets. Further considerations for work from hierarchy to conversation are addressed in Table 6.1.

Hierarchy Using Stretch and Flow Phonation

1. Establish consistent exhalation of air through rounded lips.
    (a) Use a tissue for visual feedback or a finger for kinesthetic feedback of airflow.
    (b) What does the client feel? (Whenever possible use the client's words to reflect their experience or provide framework/options for descriptors, if needed.)
        (i) Consistent airflow vs inconsistent.
        (ii) Open/easy throat vs tight/effortful throat.
2. Maintain consistent airflow and add phonation on a /u/ vowel.
    (a) Voice may vary from a whisper to having more sound depending on the client's coordination of breathing, phonation, and tension patterns (e.g., breathy vs balanced vs glottal onset).

(b) Explore variations in airflow that may create a desirable quality (breathy vs non-breathy).
(c) Begin with sustained phonation (use glides and/or sirens as an option to improve ease of coordination).

  (i) Notice the pitch that is produced and experiment on different sustained pitches moving toward the target pitch range.

(d) Expand to glides and sirens.

  (i) Continue to be aware of exploring the target pitch range.

(e) Check in with the feeling and the sound.

  (i) Is the /u/ as easy as exhaling in isolation? Can the voice feel the same as blowing?
  (ii) Where do you feel the sound (could be an opportunity to incorporate resonance work)?
  (iii) How does it sound?

    1. Smooth, rough, breathy, etc.
    2. Is it in a pitch range that is comfortable and aligning with goals?

3. Use the /u/ vowel into words, phrases, and sentences.

   (a) Stretch out the vowels and maintain airflow.

     (i) Work in the target pitch range.
     (ii) Explore intonation patterns.
     (iii) Chanting on one pitch or a combination of pitches may be a useful tool at this time in achieving pitch awareness, control, and consistency.

   (b) Begin to reduce stretch and balanced airflow while maintaining ease, quality, and pitch.

4. Use the /u/ vowel into reading.

   (a) Maintain ease, quality, and pitch.

5. Use the /u/ vowel into dialogue (Q and A and conversation).

   (a) Maintain ease, quality, and pitch.

*Steps may be skipped and do not have to be approached sequentially if not needed to achieve consistency and/or carryover. Consider moving back and forth between steps as needed.

It should be considered that using a hierarchical approach to establish coordinated phonatory airflow may not be necessary for some individuals during gender affirming voice work. Conversation training therapy (CTT) works to achieve an efficient voice with balanced phonatory airflow and to increase vocal awareness exclusively in the context of conversational speech with client-directed topics [21]. There are six primary tenets that can be used as needed or in any order required to achieve therapy goals. The tenets include "clear speech, auditory/kinesthetic awareness, rapport building, negative practice, basic training gestures, and prosody." The use of basic training gestures requires sustaining certain consonants (e.g., ʃ, j, f, v, s, z, m, n) to increase the awareness and sensations of sound energy or vibration in the mouth [21]. With these basic training gestures, airflow can be targeted as well as pitch.

CTT has recently been examined in the context of gender affirming voice work with transgender women. In this study, CTT was modified to include more direct exploration and work on pitch with five transgender women who had not previously undergone voice training. The results showed some increase in pitch across participants after five sessions of weekly therapy. The most promising results however were the relationship between self-perception of voice femininity and ratings of voice satisfaction [22]. Further research is required in this area to increase our understanding of the efficacy of CTT for gender affirming voice care, and this is a step forward in promoting evidence-based practice for those seeking gender affirmative voice care.

Pitfalls When Working with Flow Phonation

Optimizing the coordination of breathing and phonation with flow phonation can be quite helpful to achieve a voice that is gender congruent. However, for some, the use of flow phonation can result in a breathy voice that is imbalanced and without dynamic intensity or pitch change, which may not be desirable. Some may perceive this as "losing power" in the sense of reduced vocal intensity but also in the sense of vocal presence within a room or conversation. It has been shown that women after often interrupted or talked over in situations that they are outnumbered by men [23]. Anecdotally, a breathy quality without dynamic change may feel as though it contributes to these societal patterns. During voice exploration, when patterns are identified as less desirable or suboptimal, it can be an opportunity to empower the client to observe and note their volitional control over voice production and decision-making. In addition, it can be used in the form of negative practice to contrast what is desired and what may be avoided. Ultimately, if the desired voice results are not being achieved with flow phonation, another technique may be the next best option. It is important to ensure that voice work, no matter the technique, does not result in a sense of disempowerment but quite the opposite.

While this chapter focuses on the technical aspects of voice production in the forms of flow phonation, these are only one part of the therapy process that will likely include counseling, education, meta-therapy [24], and exploration regarding the connection between identity and voice, to name a few. These aspects of therapy may be explored to varying degrees based on the comfort of the treatment-seeking individual and the experience of the treating clinician. With this, it is important to seek specialized and culturally responsive care to address the multi-dimensional aspects of gender affirming voice care.

Practice and Maintenance

There is little evidence in the current literature to provide guidance on the frequency and duration of vocal practice nor the long-term outcomes of gender affirming voice therapy. To move toward implementing voice and communication techniques into daily speaking, the technical aspects of voice production must be addressed. With this, frequent, short periods of vocal practice are ideal. They offer multiple opportunities to interrupt habitual patterns, to "reset" the voice closer to the "goal voice," and to connect with new voice use patterns. In the early part of voice therapy, daily practice recommendations may include:

1. Morning: 5–10 min.
   (a) Find the "goal voice" using established techniques.
   (b) Identify vocal goals for the day.
2. Practice a few times in the middle of the day for 2–3 min each time.
   (a) Observe where the voice is and "reset" as needed.
   (b) Reconnect with daily vocal goals.
3. Evening: 5–10 min.
   (a) More repetitions with "goal voice" using established techniques.
   (b) Reflect/observe patterns from the day.

It is important to focus on the positive aspects of self-awareness and work to solidify the established skills to increase success moving forward. As therapy progresses and less formal practice is needed to find the "goal voice," periods of resetting the voice and using the techniques in day-to-day speaking may become the primary form of practice. Application of the techniques in day-to-day talking often begins as a mindful decision, although with practice and regular application finding the "goal voice" will likely begin to happen with less active thought and become more habitual.

Gelfer and Tice [25] assessed therapy outcomes with transgender women comparing listener perception of femininity before, immediately after, and the 15 months following an 8-week voice therapy program. Femininity was rated higher immediately post treatment than 15 months later, and both ratings were higher than pretreatment. While the methods used for this study could be debated, with voice therapy perceptions of femininity were impacted in a positive way, and some long-term effects were noted. However, given the reduction in perceived femininity over time, these findings may highlight the need for a voice maintenance program.

Regarding maintenance, each person is different. Some people will require continued daily practice after voice therapy has drawn to a close, while others may have integrated the new patterns and require minimal vocal attention. In either case, regular vocal check-ins can be useful for self-awareness, self-monitoring, and from a vocal health perspective. For example, scheduling a vocal check-in each Monday morning on the drive to work could be useful. During this vocal check-in, previously established voice exercises (e.g., SnF) are revisited. Observations are made regarding (1) how the voice feels and (2) how the voice sounds. Based on the observations, the person may decide their voice feels great or that resuming practice may be helpful to reconnect with their voice and maintain their vocal goals. Further work is required in this area to understand, from a research perspective, what is needed for efficacious practice and maintenance. For now, and even when the research catches up to our clinical work, we should continue to respond to each individual and modify exercises and vocal routines to meet their unique goals.

Conclusion

Focusing on the coordination of breathing and phonation during voice production is one of the hallmarks of voice work. Breath is the power source for the voice, and with this it is the foundation for altering other aspects of voice production including pitch, resonance, intonation, and intensity which are important variables that may be targeted during gender affirming voice care. Vocal techniques focused on airflow, including stretch and flow phonation, flow phonation, and semi-occluded vocal tract exercises, can be used as tools for exploration on a path to achieve a gender affirmative voice: a voice that the treatment-seeking person connects with and identifies as their own. Ultimately, as clinicians, it is our responsibility to share these tools and guide exploration to help each person meet their individual voice goals.

References

1. Gauffin J, Sundberg J. Spectral correlates of glottal voice source wave- form characteristics. J Speech Hear Res. 1989;32:556–65. https://doi.org/10.1044/jshr.3203.556.
2. Patel RR, Sundberg J, Gill B, Lã FMB. Glottal airflow and glottal area waveform characteristics of flow phonation in untrained vocally healthy adults. J Voice. 2020;36(1):140.e1–140.e21. https://doi.org/10.1016/j.jvoice.2020.07.037.
3. Stone RE, Casteel RL. Intervention in non-organically based dysphonia. New York: C.C. Thomas Co.; 1982.
4. Watts CR, Diviney SS, Hamilton A, Toles L, Childs L, Mau T. The effect of stretch-and-flow voice therapy on measures of vocal function and handicap. J Voice. 2015a;29(2):191–9. https://doi.org/10.1016/j.jvoice.2014.05.008.
5. Watts CR, Hamilton A, Toles L, Childs L, Mau T. A randomized controlled trial of stretch-and-flow voice therapy for muscle tension dysphonia. Laryngoscope. 2015b June;125(6):1420–5. https://doi.org/10.1002/lary.25155.
6. Watts CR, Hamilton A, Toles L, Childs L, Mau T. Intervention outcomes of two treatments for muscle tension dysphonia: a randomized controlled trial. J Speech Lang Hear Res. 2019;62(2):272–82. https://doi.org/10.1044/2018_JSLHR-S-18-0118.
7. Gartner-Schmidt J. Flow phonation. In: Stemple JC, Hapner ER, editors. Voice therapy: clinical case studies. 4th ed. San Diego, CA: Plural Publishing; 2014.
8. Titze IR. Voice training and therapy with a semi- occluded vocal tract: Rationale and scientific underpinnings. J Speech Lang Hear Res. 2006;49:448–59.

9. Titze IR, Finnegan E, Laukkanen A-M, Jaiswal S. Raising lung pressure and pitch in vocal warm-ups: the use of flow-resistant straws. J Sing. 2002;58:329–38.
10. Kapsner-Smith MR, Hunter EJ, Kirkham K, Cox K, Titze IR. A randomized controlled trial of two semi-occluded vocal tract voice therapy protocols. J Speech Lang Hear Res. 2015;58(3):535–49. https://doi.org/10.1044/2015_JSLHR-S-13-0231.
11. Titze IR, Laukkanen AM. Can vocal economy in phonation be increased with an artificially lengthened vocal tract? A computer modeling study. Logoped Phoniatr Vocol. 2007;32:147–56.
12. Casado JC, O'Connor C, Angulo MS, Adrián JA. Wendler glottoplasty and voice-therapy in male-to-female transsexuals: results in pre and post-surgery assessment. Acta Otorrinolaringol Esp. 2016;67(2):83–92.
13. Gorham-Rowan M, Morris R. Aerodynamic analysis of male-to-female transgender voice. J Voice Off J Voice Found. 2006;20(2):251–62.
14. Oates J, Dacakis G. Transgender voice and communication: research evidence underpinning voice intervention for male-to-female transsexual women. Perspect Voice Voice Disord. 2015;25(2):48.
15. Hillman RE, Holmberg EB, Perkell JS, et al. Objective assessment of vocal hyperfunction: an experimental framework and initial results. J Speech Lang Hear Res. 1989;32:373–92. https://doi.org/10.1044/jshr.3202.373.
16. Gartner-Schmidt J. Flow phonation. In: Behrman A, Haskel J, editors. Exercises for voice therapy. 3rd ed. San Diego, CA: Plural Publishing; 2020.
17. Fadel CB, Dassie-Leite AP, Santos RS, Santos CG Jr, Dias CA, Sartori DJ. Immediate effects of the semi-occluded vocal tract exercise with LaxVox® tube in singers. Codas. 2016;28(5):618–24. Portuguese, English. https://doi.org/10.1590/2317-1782/20162015168.
18. Mills M, Stoneham G. The voice book for trans and non-binary people. London: Jessica Kingsley Publishers; 2017.
19. Jackson Hearns L, Kremer B. The singing teacher's guide to transgender voice. San Diego, CA: Plural Publishing; 2018.
20. Titze I, Verdolini K. Vocology: The Science and Practice of Voice Habilitation. Salt Lake City: National Center for Voice & Speech; 2012.
21. Gartner-Schmidt J, Gherson S, Hapner ER, Muckala J, Roth D, Schneider S, Gillespie AI. The development of conversation training therapy: a concept paper. J Voice. 2016;5:563–73. https://doi.org/10.1016/j.jvoice.2015.06.007.
22. Peck Eng M, Schneider SL, Sundarrajan A. Conversation training therapy to target voice and communication for trans. Women presented at the 2021 Annual Symposium: Care for the Professional Voice, Philadelphia, PA. 2021
23. Karpowitz C, Mendelberg T, Sharker L. Gender inequality in deliberative participation. Am Polit Sci Rev. 2012;106(3):533–47. https://doi.org/10.1017/S0003055412000329.
24. Helou LB, Gartner-Schmidt JL, Hapner ER, Schneider SL, Van Stan JH. Mapping metatherapy in voice interventions onto the rehabilitation treatment specification system. Semin Speech Lang. 2021;42(1):5–18. https://doi.org/10.1055/s-0040-1722756.
25. Gelfer MP, Tice RM. Perceptual and acoustic outcomes of voice therapy for male-to-female transgender individuals immediately after therapy and 15 months later. J Voice. 2013;27(3):335–47. https://doi.org/10.1016/j.jvoice.2012.07.009.

Chapter 7
Resonant Voice Care

Tina Babajanians

Introduction

Resonant voice therapy is a familiar concept to speech-language pathologists and voice clinicians. Clinicians target resonant strategies in cases of hypernasality, hyponasality, tone focus, or when rehabilitating an injured voice [1]. Resonant voice therapy uses a continuum of oral and nasal vibratory sensations to promote efficient phonation, building from basic speech gestures through conversational speech. The goal is to achieve the strongest, "cleanest" possible voice with the least effort and impact between the vocal folds; this ultimately minimizes the likelihood of injury and maximizes the likelihood of vocal health [2]. One of the most well-known resonant voice programs is Lessac–Madsen Resonant Voice Therapy (LMRVT) that uses a combination of vocal hygiene efforts and a structured resonance hierarchy to rehabilitate resonance and voice.

Resonance is defined as the filter function of the vocal tract on the sound wave produced by the larynx [3]. When thinking about working on resonant voice with transgender and gender nonconforming (TGNC) clients, it is important to note that this is taking a traditional voice therapy technique and using it in a habilitative context. This is not the treatment of a disordered or injured voice; it is an elective service to facilitate a more gender-congruent voice. In the case of clients seeking a more femininely perceived voice across the gender spectrum, there is evidence to support that resonance work and vowel modification can be beneficial.

T. Babajanians (✉)
Newport Beach, CA, USA
e-mail: tina@thevoicestylist.com; https://www.thevoicestylist.com

M. S. Courey et al. (eds.), *Voice and Communication in Transgender and Gender Diverse Individuals*, https://doi.org/10.1007/978-3-031-24632-6_7

Background

In 1977, a single-case study was presented at the ASHA Convention in Chicago on therapeutic interventions for transfeminine clients [4]. This was the first published work on this subject, and since then a steady body of research has emerged. The current evidence seeks to demonstrate that resonance and vowel modification are reliable methods of intervention.

Oates and Dacakis [5] discuss that there are consistent differences between cismale and cisfemale resonance: average formant frequencies of cisfemale voices are approximately 20% higher than cismales, most formant bandwidths are wider for cisfemales, and amplitudes of most formants are lower for cisfemales compared to cismales. According to research, vocal tract resonance characteristics are explained by the acoustic theory of vowels. This states that vowel formant frequencies are determined by a combination of physical vocal tract characteristics including cavity size, shape, and mass [6]. The first (F1), second (F2), and third (F3) formants of the vocal tract are typically calculated to measure the impact of the vocal tract filter on the voice. F1 and F2 determine the vowel identity and quality, and all three vowel formants reflect the overall length of the vocal tract [7].

"The Effect of Formant Biofeedback on the Feminization of Voice in Transgender Women" [8] investigated F2 frequency during word production. They also looked at using biofeedback to manipulate F2 to match a target formant frequency typical of a cisgender female and to determine its correspondence with feminine speech perception. The results determined that participants were able to manipulate the height of F2 using visual and acoustic biofeedback. These higher F2 values were associated with higher ratings of perceived femininity of speech.

The specific use of resonance and vowel formants with transgender and gender nonconforming individuals reveals that a high front vowel /i/ may lead to an increased perception of feminine sound in speech [1]. The use of lip spreading and forward tongue carriage can increase the vowel formant frequency values of transfeminine clients [7]. The research has concluded that following oral resonance work there was a general increase in vowel formant frequency values (F1, F2, and F3) for all vowels (/i/, /a/, and /ʊ/) with the ten transgender female participants. This increase was statistically significant for F1 values of /a/ and /ʊ/), F2 values of /a/, and F3 values for all three vowels [7].

The overall evidence supports targeting resonance and vowel modification as one component of achieving a more femininely perceived voice. In general, these strategies may target forward resonance and increasing formant frequencies, but it should be noted that not all individuals will desire a forward resonance when modifying their voice to align with their gender identity. Future studies need to include TGNC individuals in their populations. Studies should also take strong consideration of societal constructs of gender and gender perception over time [9]. The TGNC community should be central in defining outcomes.

Resonance Considerations with Transgender and Gender Nonconforming Individuals

An alignment of the client's personal voice goals and clinician expertise is the foundation for making progress. The individual's satisfaction determines successful outcomes. Clinicians must set aside expectations, biases, and data based on cis-heteronormative standards in order to serve from a place of cultural competency and humility. Developing goals and objectives that are client-led and functional for real-world outcomes is critical. Allow the individual to state goals in colloquial and self-identified terms. *Client-stated goal: "I want to have a voice that is sensual and husky."* Consider how resonance and other strategies can support the stated goal. There are evidence-based recommendations, for instance, Oates and Dacakis [10] suggest targeting a fundamental frequency of at least 155 Hz while attempting to increase formant frequencies (alter resonance) as one realistic goal to consider. While the evidence does provide some framework that may be relevant to specific clients, it is essential to reference evidence-based norms with caution so as not to impose preprogrammed societal norms on the individual and their gender experience.

Individuals seek out gender voice services at different points in their transition. Their level of familiarity, experience, and understanding of their desired outcome will vary by individual. Client education is a fundamental component of successful long-term therapy. Each individual presents with varying levels of knowledge and experience. It may be helpful to inquire from where they obtained their information (e.g., YouTube, Reddit, previous therapy, etc.). Establishing baseline comprehension can improve awareness of resonance.

Resonance is one piece of a dynamic vocal experience. When integrated into a well-balanced approach, resonance targets can facilitate vocal flexibility and provide tools for an increasingly gender-aligned voice.

Techniques to Facilitate Forward Resonance

Resonant voice therapy and vowel formant modifications are the primary approaches to achieving forward resonance and facilitating a gender-congruent voice, especially in the case of voice feminization [1]. Resonance, tone, and vowel-shaping strategies are utilized from simple tasks to conversational speech. Exploration of stimulability will demonstrate where the individual is successful and how to progress through speech tasks [11, 12].

First, identify baseline resonance. Working to discover the baseline production of resonance and then progressing to manipulation of that resonance begin to reveal what the person is capable of producing. Exploring the hierarchy will demonstrate the individual's ability to produce the target resonance at various levels of speech complexity. Frequent "check-ins" allow the client to ask questions and make suggestions for what they think does or does not work, ultimately identifying strategies that create meaningful change.

From Structured Tasks to Generalization

Begin with discrimination tasks to identify the difference between forward-focused, posterior tone ("throat") focus, and "chest" resonance. It can be helpful to demonstrate exaggerated clinician models. Chest resonance is often accessed by lowering the jaw and base of the tongue and creating a larger oral cavity. The resulting sensation of resonance is felt closer to the chest [13]. Alternatively, forward-focused resonance can be accessed by forward tongue carriage, lip spreading, and creating a smaller oral cavity. Posterior tone focus is usually accompanied by a vocal strain pattern characterized by reduced airflow and increased perilaryngeal muscle tension. Chest resonance is typically associated with the perception of masculine speech whereas forward-focused resonance is associated with the perception of feminine speech. Posterior tone focus may be associated with either masculine or feminine speech, but it is important to note that this manner of speaking may be vocally fatiguing and not sustainable. It is essential to ask the client what they hear and feel to determine what resonance patterns along the continuum are congruent to the individual's goals.

Resonant Hum

Next, introduce simple isolated hums to target sensations and to begin to feel forward resonance. Research has demonstrated that /m/ promotes oral resonance and helps the individual sense vibrations in the oral cavity [14]. Biofeedback can be achieved by placing fingers gently on either side of the nose or by cupping hands over the nose and mouth while humming. Tasks should progress from simple to complex [12]. To support perceptual–motor learning, instructions should be given to "feel" for resonance. Efforts should be focused on attempting to move vibratory sensations upward and forward into the "mask" or oral and nasal space of the face. It can be helpful to explore how altering lip, tongue, and jaw posture within the hum affects sensation of resonance. Some clinicians will use chewing movements, smiling vs. not, forward tongue vs. not, and open jaw vs. closed while humming [15]. The key is exploration.

Once the client has shown they are stimulable for a forward resonance on an isolated hum, the clinician can begin training resonant voice in speech tasks. Evidence of the speech hierarchy applied to voice treatment was demonstrated by Gelfer in her article, "Voice Treatment for the Male-to-Female Transgendered Client." In her research, she concludes that behavioral change can be obtained by selecting appropriate targets and habituating the voice through chanting, world level, phrase level, sentence level, and connected speech. She specifically discusses target pitch habituation with the use of /m/ and high vowels; however this chapter will focus on the resonance components of her research [14].

Transition to Speaking Voice

Transitioning to working on speaking voice can begin by working through a series of /m/ + vowel pairing. It is not unusual for this task to be initially difficult. The first several trials might induce strain or inconsistent resonance when the hum moves to the vowel. If that occurs, remind the client to relax the upper body, breathe, find the resonant hum, and maintain the placement as they slowly move into the CV blend. When teaching vowel modification as a part of resonance, it can help to exaggerate the production of each vowel. As the client becomes proficient with the high vowel /i/, it is useful to explore all vowel productions with different tongue and lip postures to find and generalize the resonance that is most congruent to their goals.

Once stability is established in producing forward resonance in CV blends, then transition to single-syllable word lists. In research by Hirsch, she states that the use of nasal consonants /m, n, and ng/ in sentences results in a higher resonance as they are produced with less articulatory contact and tension [16]. Move through the hierarchy, from introducing short phrases to sentences and eventually into conversational speech. Many of the previously mentioned cues for exploration will apply to all levels of the hierarchy. At the conversational level, it can be useful to use "mhm" as a vocal reset, which reminds the client of their resonance target.

It is possible that the client may be successful at one level of the resonance hierarchy but not at another. Return to tasks that are successful to build confidence and check in with the individual. Ask questions to facilitate conversations surrounding the voice, resonance, and aim to determine how best to support them.

As proficiency increases continue to shape sessions to allow for the use of the optimal resonance and voice in real-life contexts. Strategies suggested by Davies et al. include practicing words that are a part of typical conversation, engaging in role plays suggested by the client, and experimenting with emotional intensity in conversation [3, 17]. These real-world tasks promote carryover of skills into everyday life.

Hierarchy of Tasks for Forward Resonance

1. Introduce resonant hum.
   - (a) Promote client awareness of oral/nasal resonance.
     - (i) Cue an easy breath and hum on "mmm."
     - (ii) Gently place fingers on either side of the nose, or cup nose and mouth while humming to sense vibrations.
     - (iii) Trial chewing movements, smiling vs. not, forward tongue vs. not, and open jaw vs. closed while humming.
2. Expand the resonant hum.
   - (a) Produce varied productions of the hum.

 (i) Use varying lengths and intonations of humming and "hmm – hmm."
 (ii) Humming up and down the scale to explore range.

 (b) Produce forward resonance in consonant + vowel (CV) pairing.

 (i) Can trial single production and repeated chanted syllables.

 - /mi/
 - /ma/
 - /mu/

3. Produce resonance in single-syllable words with /m/ and /n/ focus.

 (a) For example, moon, mean, main, and mine.
 (b) Use high vowels to encourage high tongue position.
 (c) Lip spreading.
 (d) Tongue advancement.
 (e) Client progress and satisfaction check-in.

 (i) Understanding of resonance.
 (ii) Approval of the voice quality.
 (iii) Ease of production.

4. Produce forward resonance in short phrases and sentences.

 (a) For example, monday morning in May, more mountain memories, Mom made me mash my M&Ms.

5. Generalization: produce forward resonance in short conversations and role play.

 (a) Target words that are part of daily conversation.
 (b) Focus on topics related to the client's life.
 (c) Utilize "mhm" as a vocal reset in conversation.
 (d) Engaging in role plays suggested by client to match real-life situations.
 (e) Sentences expressing feelings and emotions.
 (f) Mindful practice outside the clinic setting in a variety of real-life settings.

These steps can be worked through as a hierarchy and in a cyclical approach to revisit successful productions. The hierarchy and all of the steps do not necessarily have to be completed strictly in order as long as the individual is supported and set up for success.

Practice and Maintenance Considerations

Repetition is paramount to motor learning and achieving a gender-congruent voice that is generalized to their everyday life. According to Adler et al., there is no singular way to develop skill carryover and determine readiness for discharge with transgender clients (411). Davies states in her research that individuals not only need to generalize new skills from the clinic into daily contexts, but they also have the added challenge of aligning speech and communication to their stage of transition and their own sense of gender identity (68). Further research is necessary to provide direction on recommendations for treatment as well as daily practice. It has been anecdotally demonstrated that the individuals who participate in a daily vocal routine yield improved results.

Home practice should be reasonable and easily incorporated into the individual's life. Initial recommendations typically include short and consistent practice sessions which target the relevant goals addressed in the session that week. For example, if the session focused on producing a forward resonance at the phrase level, home practice may target repetition of these techniques for approximately 15 minutes each day, broken into 5-min periods spread throughout the day. Beginning the day with a resonance warm up also helps orient the individual toward a more forward resonance. As the sessions go on, these foundational resonance skills are established and expanded to a variety of communication contexts. The home practice and generalization strategies should reflect the client's current abilities and be consistent with their individual goals for a gender-congruent voice.

Pitfalls When Working with Resonance

Shaping a forward-focused resonance and enhancing the use of high vowel formants present a unique challenge in that it is an abstract concept that can be difficult to demonstrate [14]. Another challenge when targeting resonance is that some clients may experience muscle tension, strain, and fatigue. This may be associated with their habitual speaking patterns, the adjustments they are making in their vocal tract, and the repetitive nature of hierarchical tasks, or it may be simultaneous changes in pitch that contribute to a "high and tight" sensation in the voice. It is important to monitor and address these symptoms as they appear, given a strained or tense voice is not sustainable for most clients. Particularly in repetitive tasks, it can be useful to take breaks and use relaxing exercises. This may include respiratory techniques focused on abdominal breathing, SOVT exercises such as tongue or lip trills to re-balance the subsystems of voice, tongue tension reduction strategies, and yawn–sigh with or without a hum. Find the strategies that work for the individual client to maintain efficiency and ease in their voice.

It is essential to unlearn bias from cis-heteronormative standards and understand that there is not one way to achieve a gender-congruent resonance. For the purposes of this chapter, we are speaking in terms of general components associated with perception of feminine speech and resonance as understood by the research literature thus far. Although a framework has been defined and provided, ultimately the individual who has sought out services should define what they anticipate to be their optimal voice.

During voice sessions the individual may look to the clinician as the leader or as an external source of validation. The clinician must pay attention to this and ensure that the power and authority are always deferred back to the client. Frequently asking for client feedback and encouraging full participation are some ways to facilitate this power shift. Giving context through education and increasing vocabulary surrounding the voice (e.g., how to describe characteristics with words like husky, sultry, breathy, harsh, thin, etc.) can help center the client's perspective and facilitate their agency.

One area to address in a sensitive manner is expectation management for outcomes, speed of progress, and anticipating results. The clinician should provide education and counseling regarding the gradual process of motor learning in order to ease concern over how quickly one should be advancing. It is beneficial to highlight a client's progress through pacing out tasks, offering specific feedback, and providing meaningful home practice goals that they are held accountable to. If a client is not fully participating in the process, the clinician will need to address realistic expectations for progress, incorporate motivational interviewing and rapport building, and consider adapting goals and sessions targets.

Conclusion

In transgender and gender nonconforming voice work, the client and clinician collaborate to develop a voice that is optimal and safe. Flexibility and creativity are imperative as each client is an individual who has unique goals. While there are established hierarchies and specific strategies that may be useful to draw from, these should be used as tools to explore, not to hinder. The final and most important metric of success in resonant voice work is client satisfaction with their sound quality and ability to generalize these skills to everyday life. Keep an ongoing, open dialogue and establish strong rapport with clients. It is the clinician's responsibility to provide culturally competent and clinically sound care that facilitates the client's personal voice and communication goals.

References

1. Adler R, et al. Voice and communication therapy for the transgender/transsexual client: a comprehensive clinical guide. 2nd ed. San Diego, CA: Plural Publishing; 2012.
2. Stemple J. Voice therapy clinical studies. 2nd ed. San Diego, CA, Singular Thomson Learning; 2000.
3. Davies S, et al. Voice and communication change for gender nonconforming individuals: giving voice to the person inside. Int J Transgend. 2015;16(3):117–59. https://doi.org/10.1080/15532739.2015.1075931.
4. Kalra MA. Voice therapy with a transsexual. In: Gemme R, Wheeler C, editors. International congress on sexology. New York, NY: Plenum; 1977. p. 77–84.

5. Oates J, Dacakis G. Voice change in transsexuals. Venereology. 1997;10:178–87.
6. Coleman RO. Male and female voice quality and its relationship to vowel formant frequencies. J Speech Hear Res. 1971;14(3):565–77. https://doi.org/10.1044/jshr.1403.565.
7. Carew L, Dacakis G, Oates J. The effectiveness of oral resonance therapy on the perception of femininity of voice in male-to-female transsexuals. J Voice. 2007;21:591–603.
8. Kawitzky D, McAllister T. The effect of formant biofeedback on the feminization of voice in transgender women. J Voice. 2020;34(1):53–67. https://doi.org/10.1016/j.jvoice.2018.07.017.
9. Coleman RO. A comparison of the contributions of two voice quality characteristics to the perception of maleness and femaleness in the voice. J Speech Hear Res. 1976;19(1):168–80. https://doi.org/10.1044/jshr.1901.168.
10. Oates J, Dacakis G. Speech pathology considerations in the management of transsexualism: a review. Br J Disord Commun. 1983;18:139–51.
11. Abbott KV. Lessac-Madsen resonant voice therapy patient manual: single copy. 1st ed. San Diego, CA: Plural Publishing, Inc.; 2008.
12. Titze I, Abbott KV. Vocology the science and practice of voice habilitation. Salt Lake City, UT: National Center for Voice and Speech; 2021.
13. Sundberg J. Chest wall vibrations in singers. J Speech Lang Hear Res. 1983;26(3):329–40. https://doi.org/10.1044/jshr.2603.329.
14. Gelfer MP. Voice treatment for the male-to-female transgendered client. Am J Speech Lang Pathol. 1999;8(3):201–8. https://doi.org/10.1044/1058-0360.0803.201.
15. Stewart CF, Kling IF. University practicum for transgender voice modification: a motor learning perspective. Perspect ASHA Spec Interest Groups. 2017;2(10):102–8. https://doi.org/10.1044/persp2.sig10.102.
16. Hirsch S. Combining voice, speech science and art approaches to resonant challenges in transgender voice and communication training. Perspect ASHA Spec Interest Groups. 2017;2(10):74–82. https://doi.org/10.1044/persp2.sig10.74.
17. Davies S. The evidence behind the practice: a review of wpath suggested guidelines in transgender voice and communication. Perspect ASHA Spec Interest Groups. 2017;2(10):64–73. https://doi.org/10.1044/persp2.sig10.64.

Chapter 8
Working with Pitch in Transgender and Gender Nonconforming Voice Care

Christella Antoni

Introduction

The issue of pitch is one of the most frequently discussed aspects of the speech-language pathologist's (SLP) efforts in relation to transgender and gender diverse voice work. The issue has been around longer and to a more extensive level with regard to transfeminine voice interventions. Not least, this is due to the historically higher numbers of transgender women who present for gender-aligning voice care. Although the incidence of SLP work with transmasculine voice is increasing, the bulk of SLP undertakings has historically been with transgender women as hormone interventions do not affect an increase in their pitch or a desired change in their voice.

The broad range of transgender identities and expressions continues to evolve. This, and the personal nature of each individual's voice goals and perceptions, continues to broaden the discussion relating to pitch. It is culturally appropriate to be aware of, and promote, a broad range of possible vocal outcomes. It cannot be assumed what clients want regarding their voice; clinicians must ask and listen. "Voice and communication change is only important if it matters to the person" [1].

At the heart of all gender-aligning voice work is the overarching endeavour of working directly with client-defined goals while ensuring vocal health. The key to embarking on this joint road is the initial assessment where the client's subjective information informs our onward clinical endeavours. The range of the desired outcomes by clients drives the advancement of clinical knowledge and skills.

This chapter will discuss:

C. Antoni (✉)
Voice and Speech Services, University College London (UCL), London, UK
e-mail: voice@christellaantoni.co.uk

M. S. Courey et al. (eds.), *Voice and Communication in Transgender and Gender Diverse Individuals*, https://doi.org/10.1007/978-3-031-24632-6_8

- Fundamental frequency (pitch) and fundamental frequency range (pitch range).
- Research on pitch and pitch range therapies.
- Role/rationale for including pitch range therapies in voice modification training for transgender and gender nonconforming (TGNC) individuals.
- How to work with clients to establish starting pitch and target pitch.
- Approaches clinicians outline for pitch-based instruction with greater detail provided regarding the Antoni Method.
- Recommendations to best facilitate the client's ability to achieve their desired pitch.

Clients' personal communications have shared that those who seek voice and communication assistance, in general, highly value the guidance of a SLP. As far as possible, clinicians strive to base their work on evidence. Historically, this was not easy as it was not until the late 1970s that publications began to emerge as single-case study reports [2, 3].

Research on Pitch and Pitch Range Therapies

Research and literature reviews in female transgender voice work have increased over the years [4–9]. However, systematic research on the effectiveness of voice training for transgender women is limited. The few studies at research hierarchy level 2 appear to demonstrate the effectiveness of voice training [10, 11]. The research issue is further compounded by the individualised approach clinicians take with each client as indicated by the client's own goals for their voice. Oates reminds us that transgender women are not a homogenous population and that "This heterogeneity makes scientific control difficult and can limit the feasibility and value of randomised control trials."

Vocal behaviours are the most frequent communication intervention targets in transfeminine voice [4, 6, 9, 12]. Research findings further demonstrate that voice aspects such as fundamental frequency, fundamental frequency range and formant frequencies differ between cisfemale and cismale speakers. In addition, average fundamental frequency, upper and lower limits of fundamental frequency range and formant frequencies have been determined as voice markers of speaker gender in transgender females [13–18].

Speaking fundamental frequency (SFF) has been described as the mean or average of frequencies speaker's produce in connected speech. This can vary due to a variety of influences such as intensity, phonemic composition and message intention [19]. SFF is measured in Hertz (Hz)—the amount of vocal fold cycles per second as the vocal folds open and close. Some clinicians recommend working with semitones when measuring pitch, particularly if the clinician works with a piano, pitch pipe or tone-producing app "As Hz values do not necessarily correspond well to perceptions of pitch" [20]. Pitch matching or voice production using sung or musically played notes is not featured in Antoni Method voice modification systems for speaking voice, and thus Hertz measurement is used for voice analysis. However, each clinician works to their own preferred methods, and an awareness of both measurement systems is helpful. Access to a conversion scale of semitone and Hz values is also useful (see Appendix 1).

It is not surprising that fundamental frequency and pitch, its perceptual correlate, is the most researched aspect of voice in transgender females. Fundamental frequency and pitch range are measurable, whereas aspects such as resonance do not lend themselves easily to scientific analysis. Resonance work has perhaps a strong reliance in proprioception as well as voice placement and feeling, the latter concepts having a greater footing in artistic voice work. However, voice is a multi-dimensional phenomenon with many interrelated aspects which are difficult to fully separate; working on resonance, for example, can significantly influence pitch and vice versa.

Greene and Mathieson describe the average SFF in cismales to be 128 Hz and 225 Hz in cisfemales [21]. However, habitual voices vary greatly, from speaker to speaker, and within those variations, they may be further influenced, not least by circumstances and emotions. Age also contributes to pitch with pitch increases associated with older males, while some pitch lowering is noted in older females as the vocal folds thicken slightly with age [22]. Thus, while higher average SFF has been reported in younger females between 20 and 29 years [23], women in their 30 s, 40 s and 50 s are reported to be below 200 Hz [19].

Studies have shown that voices can be perceived as female by listeners at a speaking fundamental frequency around 155 Hz–160 Hz [17, 18]. Literature reviews suggest that SFF above 140 Hz and moving towards the cisfemale range of 180 Hz–220 Hz is indicated for listener perception of female voice [4, 9, 24]. This considerable range overlap provides multiple paths forward regarding available gender-acceptable pitch for TGNC individuals.

Role/Rationale for the Use of Pitch Range Therapies in Voice Modification Training with TGNC Individuals

A review of the literature by McNeil found that "speech and language therapy is successful at creating an acceptable fundamental frequency in transgender patients" [25]. Nevertheless, available structured protocols and programmes for working directly with pitch and pitch range are lacking. General frameworks usually outline a broad range of interventions but are limited in specific technique description.

Pitch range therapies with TGNC individuals can be centred in the treatment outcomes sought by clients and the available evidence. The growth of transgender and gender diverse voice services around the world indicates the consistent number increase of individuals seeking professional guidance regarding voice and communication. This growth is true for both public funded health systems in Europe, including Sweden and the UK's National Health Service (NHS) and US services where the client's treatment may be funded by private health insurance. A rapid growth of demand and referrals is a frequent finding for newer established services [26]. Perhaps more significantly, in private practice services internationally, where clients self-fund their treatment and the majority of clients self-refer, service demand is also persistently high.

Clients present to services with their own respective voice goals. A percentage of caseload clients do not require the treatment outcome of persistent perception of a female speaker. This group may include individuals who identify anywhere along the gender spectrum, such as nonbinary or genderfluid, and the percentage may well increase over time. For these clients, a variety of treatment targets may be appropriate. However, transgender women seeking the treatment outcome of a voice that is consistently perceived as female have historically remained the larger caseload percentage in the majority of TGNC voice services. For these individuals, a comprehensive approach to voice feminization and typically a longer treatment intervention period are usually required.

Gender-neutral average pitch, from approximately 140 Hz to 160 Hz, may be a useful goal for nonbinary clients if this is aligning with the voice they are aiming for. This goal is typically quicker to achieve and sustain. It can bring social comfort to individuals who do not wish for a categorically male or female voice presentation. For those clients desiring a consistently female voice presentation, targeting the average SFF above 160 Hz is often indicated.

Determining with Patients, Which Pitch to Begin with and/or Target, and Methods to Achieve This

During the initial evaluation session, the client's baseline pitch measures for both reading and spontaneous speech are gathered via voice recordings. This also allows the SLP to make a perceptual analysis of the client's voice quality and to grade any presenting dysphonia. The latter will influence the initial treatment and exercises since it is recommended that dysphonia is eliminated as soon as possible. If dysphonia is noted, and the client has not been referred by ENT, a referral for a laryngeal exam is required.

Forward resonance exercises involving the sound /m/ are routinely used in voice remediation programmes [27, 28]. This type of semi-occluded vocal tract exercise has been found to be beneficial for reduction of muscle tension dysphonia (MTD) and can be easily adapted to work with transfeminine of TGNC vocal resonance. In addition, increasing oro-facial resonance is likely to assist with beginning pitch elevation work since "high pitch is not necessarily the result of high frequency but may be caused by the acoustic characteristics imparted to the voice by the supraglottic tract" [21].

Antoni Method Approach and Protocol for Transfeminine and TGNC Work [The Antoni Method Protocol Is Outlined in Appendix 2]

Exercise 1: Resonance and Pitch Contrast Exercise

Asking new clients to make the /m-hmm/ sound as if in agreement in their usual (starting) pitch helps establish awareness of their current pitch and often how they produce voice. For example, the sound can often be pressed or constricted in the throat, rather than containing a balance of facial resonance. A recommended approach is outlined below:

- Demonstrate the /m-hmm/ sound, and then ask the client to repeat while placing two fingers lightly first on one side of their nose and then the other, to help them feel vibrations.
- The client can be asked to repeat the /m-hmm/ sound in a pitch slightly higher than their own usual pitch. Hearing a higher pitch demonstrated by the clinician will assist clients to do this although the goal in the Antoni Method is not for the client to match the pitch demonstrated by the clinician but rather for the client to find a slightly higher pitch than their own starting pitch using the /m-hmm/ sound (audio-visual demonstration of forward resonance exercises as presented to clients can be viewed on the Christella VoiceUp app (Speech Tools Ltd.) [29].

This repetition of /m-hmm/ as a starting exercise can jointly target both forward resonance and higher pitch experimentation. In cases where clients produce a very high-pitched or falsetto voice when practising this combined resonance and pitch exercise, tension often plays a key role. Feeling nervous can be a prevalent feature of the initial sessions together with a general lack of awareness regarding gender-acceptable pitch range. It may be the case that clients feel the higher the pitch, the more female the voice will sound, but sharing the range of acceptable pitch for female voice identification will begin to increase client openness to what is possible. It can also bring a sense of relief to clients as using a higher pitch very early in the voice modification process can sometimes feel physically challenging with an increased risk of vocal hyperfunction and more commonly emotional discomfort.

Once a stable, clear /m-hmm/ sound at a pitch above the client's usual pitch has been achieved, this pitch can be measured and used as a target starting pitch. Alternatively, progressing to the next level of adding vowel sounds to /m/ can continue without pitch measurement to further allow the client to develop comfort in finding this new voice placement. More commonly the latter method is used avoiding too much voice measurement in the initial treatment stage as early experiential practice has proved to be the most valuable approach, anecdotally. Once adding vowel sounds has been practised, for example, /ma/, /me/, /my/, /moh/, and /moo/, pitch measurement can be made to provide guidance to the client although not essential—gaining some familiarity trying the technique is the main goal at this point, and measuring pitch once longer real-word utterances have been practised is often more useful.

Antoni Approach describes voice development and pitch change as a staged process.

The end of stage 1 goals (after approximately four treatment sessions) is that the client is able to achieve a gender-neutral average pitch (approx. 140 Hz–160 Hz) in reading voice. Typically, clients will achieve a lower average pitch in their extemporaneous speech sample. Modifying the spontaneous speaking voice is a greater challenge for all voice clients, since more thought is required for generating speech rather than reading or repeating, particularly in early stages of treatment; informing clients that this is normal helps them accept the staged process of voice change. Repeat audio recordings of reading and speech samples are advised after approximately four treatment sessions and compared with baseline recordings.

The end of stage 1 recordings can be a very satisfying moment of the treatment process. At least some levels of audio perceptual changes are the norm at his juncture, usually supported by the objective voice measures of pitch. Achieving gender-neutral average pitch in reading is a strong indicator of habitual gender-neutral voice potential if this is the client's goal. In the majority of cases, it is also a good prognostic indicator for extending the average pitch above 160 Hz for client's seeking a female voice outcome from treatment. To facilitate the latter, additional exercises to build vocal stamina and assist generalisation are usually required.

It is also during stage 1 of transfeminine voice work that intonation and mild vowel lengthening are introduced, typically included into the second treatment session. As pitch and intonation are heavily connected aspects of voice, this allows for key feminine voice aspects to be integrated early into the process which helps expedite progress. Intonation can be defined as "a change in frequency with or without interruption of phonation, of at least two semitones" [13]. Studies report that cis-females use more pitch variability and upward shifts in pitch ([13, 30]).

It is unrealistic and unnecessary for clients to achieve a specific SFF at all times. All individuals have a speaking pitch range within which a most commonly occurring frequency prevails. For this reason, measuring the modal pitch (most commonly occurring frequency) is recommended when possible (e.g., using electrolaryngology rather than measuring the average pitch which can be skewed by random low or high utterances. However, more often than not, the modal and the average pitches are closely aligned. The total or maximum phonational frequency range is not as important as establishing a comfortable conversational pitch range. A variability of approximately 12 semitones has been recommended for transfeminine voice, plus/minus one semitone area around the given SFF: "Once a client's individual SFF has been established within the gender acceptable or feminine speaking range" [20]. "Based on the client's vocal potential, any variation of the division of the semitone range is possible (e.g., 8 above and 4 below)." For example, using a 12-semitone conversational range around a target SFF of 180 Hz would result in an upper limit target of 247 Hz and a lower target limit of 131 Hz [20].

Specific Techniques for Pitch-Based Instruction

An awareness of pitch range based on the average SFF is not only important for the clinician but is also helpful for clients to assist their home practice monitoring using pitch-measuring software and apps. It is not necessary to take measurements of pitch in every session although some clinicians may favour the latter approach. In the Antoni Method, a specific average pitch is not targeted at the outset, just the initial loose goal of achieving a gender-neutral average pitch in reading by the end of session 4. This allows the client's voice to develop and the client's ear to adjust in a less pressured and step-wise way. It also allows for flexibility in case the client's treatment goals change during the therapy process. In some cases, clients achieve an average higher pitch than this by session 4. For others, pitch increases are more gradual and generally increase further in stage 2 (approximately sessions 5–8), particularly for clients seeking female-perceived voice outcome. Ultimately, the client's SFF may well settle at an average higher pitch, e.g., 200 Hz–220 Hz (especially for some younger clients) or an average lower pitch, e.g., between 160 Hz and 200 Hz, which is often acceptable and easier for clients to achieve. This range of possible outcomes for clients wishing for female-perceived voice outcome seems to be in line with the breadth of speaking fundamental frequencies found in cisfemale voices. For this reason, targeting average female SFF is not a set goal in the Antoni Method when working with pitch.

In contrast, other clinicians have voice training systems that advocate targeting a specific pitch early in treatment such as Kathe Perez's EvaF.app. "Eva's Pitch 1 lesson trains your ear to hear the A3 pitch (220 Hz) and trains your voice to tune to that pitch." This pitch is described as an "anchoring pitch" to help clients move into the feminine pitch range. Lessons 3, 4, and 5 also focus on pitch (sound, words to phrase level, respectively) "meant to be worked together as a group, meaning that you'll spend several weeks going back and forth between these three lessons" [31]. This system has 20 lessons each worked on for 20 mins with recommendations for additional practice in between sessions.

Other clinicians do not target pitch directly. Tina Babajanians reports: "I do not emphasise pitch work, but instead try to find other access points for a feminine voice" [32]. Andrews suggests "...the pitch level is actually less important as a feminine speech marker than is pitch variability..." and continues "Feminine intonation patterns and increased vocal variety are important goals." She also emphasises the considerable overlap in the pitch range of men and women [33].

The SLT service at London's Tavistock NHS Gender Clinic states "they offer help to raise pitch to a comfortable level" as one of the aspects of transfeminine voice training they provide in "up to four one to one sessions" spaced at monthly intervals.

While outlines of general approaches to pitch work can be found, specific techniques for pitch-based instruction are more elusive. However, supralaryngeal adjustments and formant frequencies have been described as playing an influential role in the perception of female voice [10, 13, 34]. "Physiologically speaking, the articulatory positions assumed by the vocal tract determine which frequencies will be resonated" [35]. In transfeminine clients where a genderfluid pitch range has been achieved, elevated vowel formants appear to correlate with increased perception of female voice [34]. A study involving ten transgender women demonstrated that targeting forward tongue carriage and lip spread as for the vowel /i/ resulted in formant frequency changes; *F3* values increased for the vowels /a/, /i/ and /oo/, and mean *f0* increased even though pitch was not specifically targeted. The listener ratings for masculinity/femininity were mixed although both listeners and participants reported increased perception of female voice quality after treatment [36].

Tone "colour" of vowels has also been described as playing an influential role in female-perceived voice. Hirsch et al. describe the tone "colour" as moving from light to dark as vowels move from front to back. "The application of an /i/ lip configuration across vowels, especially the extended and more rounded and elongated vowels such as /u/, acts to artificially shorten the vocal tract due to lip spreading for the /i/" [35].

Lightening the Vocal Tone

Lightening the tone can also form a significant part of transfeminine voice work. Specifically, the /i/ lip and tongue posture (as for "eat") are contrasted with the /ah/ mouth and tongue posture (as for "art") to first build clients' awareness of oral postures. "However, the technique of raised back of tongue and lip spread for all vowels can prove effortful. While this technique is taught as an adjunct or support approach to vocal tone adjustment, [a] key approach is to modify the vocal tone using a thin vocal fold, non-breathy voice quality" (Working With Transgender & Gender Diverse Voice Online Course for SLT/Ps, Level 2, Teachable, 2021).

Further, the vocal tone in terms of emotional feeling also plays a significant role. In this chapter, vocal tone is referred here in the standard/lay way it tends to be referred to with regard to expressing the speaker's feelings or mood.

Emotional Tone of Voice Range

Intonation is strongly linked with emotional expression, and practising a wide range of vocal tones can be a key influencer in developing ability with pitch and voice use. This aspect of transfeminine voice work is often overlooked but anecdotally tends to lead to more voice flexibility and confidence. It can also help prevent clients becoming locked into a narrow pitch range with a uniform tone that may sound high pitched but nevertheless may not be perceived as female by listeners. Consider, for example, many different ways the word "fine" can be spoken/expressed from animated to angry. Vocal expression exercises are typically introduced in the intermediate stage of treatment once confidence has increased and additional clinician-client trust has developed.

Voice Onset Practice

An additional helpful pitch technique is voice onset practice. Practising higher pitch while encouraging lighter vocal onset for vowels, vowel onset words and phrases can help clients develop the use of thinner vocal folds. This combined with vocal expression exercises—practising a range of emotional tones of voice—assists with lightening the vocal tone.

Twang Voice Quality

As described above, supraglottic adjustments can significantly influence pitch. A narrowing and shortening of the vocal tract result in a brighter vocal tone particularly in higher pitches. Narrowing in the pharynx and aryepiglottic region produces higher formant frequencies [37]. The vocal tract postures described here are found in "Twang voice quality." "This quality works best when combined with thin vocal folds and a closed velar port" [38]. True twang voice quality does not involve constriction at the level of the larynx; the false vocal folds are retracted, eliminating the risk of vocal strain or irregularity. Vocal fold retraction can be achieved by adopting a laugh posture in the larynx [39].

Some voices are naturally brighter than others due to factors such as an individual's accent and habitual tongue posture for vowels. In addition, some increase in vocal brightness can occur naturally, during the general pitch and voice modification process. For these clients, developing twang voice quality may not feature in their therapy process. For others however, it can be a very useful technique to practise with clients. More specifically it can be used in the later stage of therapy to develop higher pitch safe voice projection skills. Many transfeminine clients are fearful of using louder volume. The traditional methods of teaching voice projection, centred in increased breath support, are generally not as effective as twang voice quality which lends itself to higher pitch and where voice amplification occurs primarily via supraglottic and oral adjustments. Clients who successfully experience achieving this technique often lose their fear of using louder volume and note the ease with which their voice can carry over space and noise. The level of twang can be adjusted according to the needs of the speaker.

The easiest way to begin tends to be with a nasal twang as for an exaggerated cat-like /meyow/, extending to nasalised vowels: /ngya/, /ngyI/, /ngyoh/ and /ngyoo/ [38]. The aim is to move from nasal twang to oral twang vowels since nasality tends to dampen the vocal tone. This can be facilitated by adopting higher tongue posture as for /y/ and extending to call out phrases such as /yes/, /hi/, /bye/ and /dinner's ready/.

Recommendations for Facilitating the Patient's Ability to Achieve the Desired Pitch

Demonstrations by the clinician can feature heavily in the initial and intermediate stages of therapy both for all key voice feminization aspects. For example, it is easier for clients to attempt intonation variation after hearing examples demonstrated by the clinician. Again, the aim is not for the client to mirror the exact intonation delivery demonstrated but rather to become sensitised to the wider scope of intonation variation availability. It is in stages 2 and 3 of the treatment process that the length and complexity of reading and spoken tasks are gradually extended. A wide variety of texts are used to practise specific voice aspects from simple rhymes to longer poems and speeches.

A completely uniform programme of voice techniques and exercises can never be provided for all clients. The more advanced in skills the practitioner is, the more exercises and techniques can be adapted, extended or even created to facilitate the client's learning and practice. In general however, with the majority of clients, key exercises and techniques are covered in the Antoni Method [the method is outlined in Appendix 2]. A summary of these is provided below:

- Resonance contrast exercise—chest vs. oro-facial.
- Pitch contrast exercise—starting habitual pitch contrasted with a slightly higher pitch.
- Lightening the vocal tone—practising /i/ tongue and lip posture and lighter vocal fold onsets.
- Intonation variation combined with mild vowel elongation, practising questions first and then extending to everyday words, rhymes and poems.
- Combining above voice aspects practising reading and speech tasks of increasing length.
- Practising a range of vocal tones including animated, relaxed, doubtful, irritated, etc.
- Different levels of voice intensity (volume), +/− twang voice quality.

The exercises and techniques used by the clinician are always important in any type of voice work, but of equal value are the therapeutic support skills employed by the therapist [40]. Advanced skills tend to come with experience and a high volume of clients. While shorter-length intervention and basic voice feminization skills can be adequate for developing gender-neutral voice presentation, advanced practitioner-level skills cannot develop if only a limited number of treatment sessions are the service norm. Very often, enhanced skills emanate from clients who possess the goal of having their voices consistently perceived as female. For the vast majority of clients and clinicians, this is a more challenging goal to reach. Female-perceived voice and pitch goals are achieved by a range of techniques and to develop exercises and therapeutic support approaches that facilitate the desired voice presentation.

Pitch cannot be practised in isolation. It is heavily linked to resonance and intonation and can be influenced by environmental context and emotional mood.

Further, therapeutic support aspects such as helping clients to desensitise to practising with the clinician and hearing their modified voice play a significant role in assisting clients to continue along their voice journeys. Sustained support is required to build clients' confidence and ability to habituate their voice. Perception vs. reality is an early consistent theme where clients hoping for a female voice outcome perceive their voice to be "too high" or sounding "too fake," and recordings are extremely helpful to assist the client's awareness that this is rarely the case.

It is also helpful to reassure clients that while the goal is a natural sounding voice, the initial steps will very likely take them outside of their comfort zone for almost all new learning processes. There are countless analogies that can be employed to assist clients through the challenges of voice work. For example, the analogy of how alien it would feel to a non-horse rider to sit on a horse for the first time and get through the first few lessons!

Although voice work with TGNC individuals can be challenging for both clients and clinicians, it is a finite process. It can be beneficial to discuss this with clients at the start of their treatment and during the process and use the analogy of learning to drive a car which involves going through a series of lessons before conscious learning becomes unconscious and no further lessons are required. These analogies and perhaps several others clinicians may employ and serve to help clients work towards their goals. What cannot be denied is the rewarding nature of this type of clinical work and the value placed upon it by our clients.

Appendix 1

Conversion table of Semitone & Hertz Values

Semitone Value	Hertz Value	Semitone Value	Hertz Value	Semitone Value	Hertz Value
C2	65	C3	130.8	C4	261.6
C#	69.30	C#	138.6	C#	277.2
D	73.43	D	146.8	D	293.7
D#	77.76	D#	155.6	D#	311.1
E	82.40	E	164.8	E	329.6
F	87.35	F	174.6	F	349.2
F#	92.50	F#	185.0	F#	370.0
G	98.03	G	196.0	G	392.0
G#	103.8	G#	207.7	G#	415.5
A	110.0	A	220.0	A	440.0
A#	116.5	A#	233.1	A#	466.2
B2	123.5	B3	247.0	B4	493.9

Source: Adapted from M.L Andrews (1999), *Manual of Voice Treatment: Paediatrics Through Geriatrics* (2nd ed.). San Diego, CA: Singular

Appendix 2

Antoni Method Treatment Protocol for TGNC voice

- A three staged process of treatment
- Audio recordings made at the start of treatment and after each stage
- Therapeutic advice and counselling support accompanies each stage of treatment
- Hierarchical tasks increasing in length, variety and complexity for both reading and speaking in each stage

TREATMENT STAGE	THERAPEUTIC ADVICE/ COUNSELLING SUPPORT EXAMPLES	TYPICAL VOICE OUTCOME STAGE
STAGE 1		
• **Baseline recordings** - Reading - Speech sample	- Desensitisation to voice - Voice acceptance at this stage	
• **Management of any Dysphonia**	- Increasing voice care - Release of tension exercises	
• **Initial exercises** - Resonance contrast exercise - Pitch contrast exercise - Intonation exercise using short questions - Vowel lengthening practicea - Short length conversation practice	- Acknowledgement of altered awareness and uncertainty re voice sound - Reassurance that spontaneous speech is more challenging	
• **End of stage 1 recordings**		- Gender-neutral pitch/voice achieved in reading - Some ability sustaining modified voice in speech
STAGE 2		
• **Intermediate level exercises** - Combining resonance, pitch Intonation, vowel lengthening in longer length reading tasks - Beginning expressive voice tone variation - Beginning volume practice - Telephone practice - Conversation practice tasks of longer length	- Encouragement to use voice in some social settings - Acknowledgement that spontaneous speech may require more practice and social comfort /experience - Encouraging a flexible voice - Telephone script role-play - Providing prompts & suggestions	- Gender-neutral to feminine in reading - Gender-neutral in speech or Gender neutral to feminine in speech - Feminine in reading & speech
• **End of stage 2 recordings**		
STAGE 3		
• **Advanced level exercises** - Reading tasks of longer length (up to one page of text)	-	
- Conversation practice involving more detail e.g. describing a holiday - Sustaining louder volume tasks	- Providing topic ideas to help client sustain on topic	
- Practising varied emotional expression e.g. using a story	- Suggestion that a little exaggeration in reading can help develop voice & general voice confidence	- Female voice when reading - Female or gender-neutral speaking voice
• **End of stage 3 recordings**		

Additional guidance

- Some individuals will achieve their goals sooner than others whilst others may benefit from additional sessions to achieve a voice that more closely aligns with their gender identity/expectations
- Social comfort, individual confidence levels, motivation for treatment and ability to practice can significantly influence the level of voice outcome
- In many cases, social comfort increases as vocal confidence increases

References

1. Antoni C. Voice, speech & language therapy. In: Bouman WP, Arcelus J, editors. The transgender handbook, a guide for transgender people, their families and professionals. New York: Nova Publishing; 2017.
2. Bralley RC, Bull GL, Gore CH, Edgerton MT. Evaluation of vocal pitch in male transsexuals. J Commun Disord. 1978;11:443–9.
3. Kalra MA. Voice training with a transsexual. Paper presented at the American Speech and Hearing Association Convention, Chicago, IL. 1977.
4. Davies S, Papp VG, Antoni C. Voice and communication change for gender nonconforming individuals: Giving voice to the person inside. Int J Transgend. 2015;16:117–59.
5. Oates JM, Dacakis G. Speech Pathology considerations in the management of transsexualism—a review. Br J Disord Commun. 1983;18:139–51.
6. Oates JM, Dacakis G. Voice change in transsexuals. Venerology. 1997;10:178–87.
7. Pickering J, Baker L. Voice and communication intervention for individuals in the transgender community: An historical perspective and review of the literature. In: Adler R, Hirsch S, Mordaunt M, editors. Voice and communication training for the transgender/transsexual client. A comprehensive guide (2nd ed., Chap1). San Diego, CA: Plural Publishing; 2012.
8. Oates JM, Dacakis G. Voice, speech and language considerations in the management of maletofemale transsexualism. Trans Sex Reassign. 1986;82–91.
9. Oates J, Dacakis G. Transgender voice and communication: research evidence underpinning voice intervention for male-to-female transsexual women. Persp Voice Voice Disord. 2015;25(2):48–58.
10. Gelfer MP, Tice RM. Perceptual and acoustic outcomes of voice therapy for male-to-female transgender individuals immediately after therapy and 15 months later. J Voice. 2013;27(3):335–47.
11. Gelfer MP, Van Dong BR. A preliminary study in the use of vocal function exercises to improve voice in male-to-female transgender clients. J Voice. 2013;27:321–34.
12. Neuman K, Welzel C. The importance of the voice in male-to-female transsexualism. J Voice. 2004;18:153–67.
13. Gelfer MP, Schofield KJ. Comparison of acoustic and perceptual measures of voice in male to female transsexuals perceived as female versus those perceived as male. J Voice. 2000;14(1):22–3.
14. Gunzburger D. Voice adaptation by transsexuals. Clin Linguist Phonet. 1989;3:163–72.
15. Gunzburger D. An acoustic analysis and some perceptual data concerning voice change in male-female trans-sexuals. Eur J Disord Commun. 1993;28:13–21.
16. Gunzburger D. Acoustic and perceptual implications of the transsexual voice. Archiv Sex Behav. 1995;24:339–48.
17. Spencer L. Speech characteristics of male-to-female transsexuals: a perceptual and acoustic study. Folia Phoniatr. 1988;40:31–42.
18. Wolfe VL, Ratusnik DL, Smith FH, Northrop GE. Intonation and fundamental frequency in male-to-female transsexuals. J Speech Hear Disord. 1990;55:43–50.
19. Colton R, Casper JK, Leonard R. Understanding voice problems. A physiological perspective for diagnosis and treatment. 3rd ed. Baltimore, MD: Lippincott Williams and Wilkins; 2006.
20. Pausewang Gelfer M, Pickering J, Mordant M. Pitch & intonation. In: Adler R, Hirsch S, Pickering J, editors. Voice and communication therapy for the transgender/gender diverse client a comprehensive clinical guide. 3rd ed. San Diego, CA: Plural Publishing; 2019. p. 191–216.
21. Greene M, Matthieson L. The voice & its disorders. 6th ed. London: Whurr Publishers; 2001.
22. Antoni C, Sandhu G. Gender dysphoria and the larynx. In: Costello D, Sandhu G, editors. Practical laryngology. Boca Raton, FL: Taylor Francis; 2016.
23. Stoicheff M. Speaking fundamental frequency characteristics of nonsmoking female adults. J Speech Hear Res. 1981;24:437–41.

24. King RS, Brown GR, McRea CR. Voice parameters that result in identification or misidentification of biological gender in male-to-female transgender veterans. Int J Transgend. 2012;13(3):117–30.
25. McNeill EJ. Management of the transgender voice. J Laryngol Otol. 2006;120(7):521–3. https://doi.org/10.1017/S0022215106001174. PMID: 16834800.
26. Lara P, Peterson G. A collaborative effort for development of a voice modification clinic for transgender individuals in a medically underserved community. Perspectives. 2018;3(14):87–94.
27. Lee L. Refocussing laryngeal tone. In: Stemple J, editor. Voice therapy: clinical studies. New York: Delmar Learning; 2000. p. 145–54.
28. Verdolini K. Lessac-Masden resonant voice therapy: sensory processing-broad practice. Pittsburgh, PA: University of Pittsburgh; 2002.
29. Speech Tools Ltd. Christella VoiceUp (Version 4.1). [Mobile version]. 2021. Accessed 29 Apr 2021.
30. Hancock A, Colton L, Douglas F. Intonation and gender perception: Applications for transgender speakers. J Voice. 2014;28:203–9.
31. VoxPop LLC. EvaF.app. (Version 3.0.6). [Mobile version]. 2021. Accessed 28 Apr 2021.
32. Babajanians T. Giving voice to gender expression. ASHA Leader. 2019;24:2.
33. Andrews ML. Manual of voice treatment, paediatrics through geriatrics. San Diego, CA: Singular Publishing; 1999.
34. Hillenbrand JM, Clark MJ. The role of f0 and formant frequencies in distinguishing the voices of men and women. Atten Percept Psychophys. 2009;71(5):1150–66.
35. Hirsch S, Pausewang-Gelfer M, Boonin J. Art and science of resonance, articulation and volume. Voice and communication therapy for the transgender/gender diverse client: A comprehensive clinical guide. 2019;217–48.
36. Carew L, Dacakis G, Oates J. The effectiveness of oral resonance therapy on the perception of femininity of voice in male-to-female transsexuals. J Voice. 2007;21(5):591–603.
37. Yanagisawa E, Estill J. The contribution of aryepiglottic constriction to "ringing" voice quality. J Voice. 1990;3:342–50.
38. Antoni C. Principles of speech and language therapy. In: Costello D, Sandhu G, editors. Practical laryngology. Boca Raton, FL: Taylor Francis; 2016.
39. Citardi M, Yanagisawawa E, Estill J. Videoendoscopic analysis of laryngeal function during laughter. Ann Otol Rhinol Laryngol. 1996;105(7):545–9.
40. Antoni C. Voice and speech training for the transgendered patient: what the otolaryngologist should know. Otolaryngol Clin North Am. 2022;55(4):749–56.

Chapter 9
Nonverbal Communication

Ali Heitzman, Libby Lavella Perfitt, and Aaron Ziegler

Nonverbal communication is broadly defined as the way we exchange information or ideas using tools other than spoken language. In addition to nonverbal vocalizations like laughing, communicating nonverbally involves sensory modalities beyond hearing and includes facial expressions, eye gaze (oculesics), physical appearance, body movements (kinetics) and posture, use of space (proxemics) and time (chronemics), and touch (haptics). There are other sensory modalities of nonverbal communication that will not be explored in this chapter such as smell (olfactory), artifacts, and environment. Linguistically meaningful visual elements such as hand motions, torso movements, and facial expressions contribute to sign languages that facilitate communication among deaf and hard-of-hearing individuals [1]. Nonverbal communication also contributes to social language (pragmatics), such as conveying turn-taking, maintaining interest, or giving context to humor and sarcasm [2]. In this chapter, the speech-language pathologist's (SLP) role in supporting clients with their nonverbal communication to promote affirming gender expression is illustrated. A safe, compassionate, and discovery-based approach to training that honors all gender identities and recognizes people of all cultures and abilities is described. The training approach allows clients the freedom to progress at their own pace, centers their preferences and goals, and ultimately provides them with an empowering experience to draw from after discharge.

A. Heitzman
Outpatient, UCLA, Los Angeles, CA, USA
e-mail: aheitzman@mednet.ucla.edu

L. Lavella Perfitt
Singuistics, Pinole, CA, USA
e-mail: libby@singuistics.com

A. Ziegler (✉)
Wellness Group for Voice, Speech, and Swallowing, LLC, Portland, OR, USA
e-mail: ziegler@wellnessgroupslp.com

M. S. Courey et al. (eds.), *Voice and Communication in Transgender and Gender Diverse Individuals*, https://doi.org/10.1007/978-3-031-24632-6_9

Rationale for and Role of Training

Gender in the realm of communication is complex. Most aspects of communication have some assumed gender roles, adopted and perpetuated by media, educational systems, cultural norms, and systemic biases, and therefore contribute to gender perception. While much attention has historically been put on voice in gender-affirming communication support, nonverbal aspects of communication play an important role in gender communicative expression and perception. Nonverbal communication has long been researched and found to be associated with gender perception in cisgender speakers [3]. Research into the role that nonverbal communication plays in gender perception for transgender and gender-expansive individuals is greatly lacking. In the limited existing research literature, nonverbal behavior appears to impact gender perception in transgender individuals as well [4, 5]. The following points outline the rationale for training nonverbal aspects of communication:

- Gendered aspects of communication are not limited exclusively to voice – specifically fundamental frequency (f_0), first and second formant frequencies (F1 and F2), and intonational contours.
- Gender perception is not limited exclusively to perceived voice and speech characteristics.
- Nonverbal aspects of communication are valuable components of communication and gender expression.

The SLP's role in gender-affirming care encompasses the provision of education and training in nonverbal communicative aspects congruent with a client's gender identity. During that process, the SLP has a responsibility to center clients in the acceptance, adaptation, and decision-making about communication and to make clients the primary agent for changing their nonverbal gender expression [6]. To that end, SLPs guide clients to make informed decisions by providing education on how people communicate – including nonverbally – in various scenarios, social circles, and situations (e.g., communicating with a close friend versus communicating with a client or communicating in person at the workplace versus communicating online with friends) as well as how gender is perceived during these communication acts. Then, clients have the option to try out various styles of communicating nonverbally (e.g., adjusting proxemics by increasing or decreasing distance or adding haptic behaviors such as touching one's hair when listening), accept or reject what they already use nonverbally in various contexts, and integrate nonverbal aspects of communication that support their expression of self. Clients may feel that a behavior resonates more with their assigned gender (e.g., excessive high five with co-workers), and they may move toward using it less while integrating a preferred behavior. In this way, the SLP provides a safe space for exploration of nonverbal communicative style, avoids reducing intricate nonverbal aspects of communication to simply masculine-feminine acts, and facilitates a client-led intervention that focuses on the client's experiences and goals.

Client goals can and should vary greatly, being unique to the individual and the lens through which they are viewing support. While some clients may be concerned with exploring and better supporting expression of their gender, other clients may come in with a goal more related to, at least initially, other's perceptions of their gender. Some clients may have goals incorporating a combination of lenses, both aligning gender expression and other's perceptions of their gender through their communication acts. For example, one client's goal with a lens focused on perception could be "I want to be gendered correctly when meeting new people at least 90% of the time." In contrast, a client focused primarily on exploring and aligning their gender expression and not necessarily concerned with how others perceive their gender could be "I want to feel more androgynous when I'm at weekly social events." Measuring goals relies on the client taking data. In the case of a goal focused on perception – and only if the client is comfortable – the client can identify opportunities to tally instances when they are perceived by others in a manner that is congruent with their gender. A client goal focused on aligning gender expression can be measured by weekly self-ratings using a gender congruence scale. Above all, goals and metrics should be developed with clients, reflecting their views and priorities to ensure support is truly client centered.

Research on Nonverbal Communication and Gender Expression

The following overview summarizes published research on nonverbal communication and gender expression. Research currently in publication is limited and frequently outdated, often generalizing findings from a Western perspective and not considering external influences. Current research into nonverbal communication and gender does not intentionally include transgender and gender-expansive participants, nor does it include non-heterosexual participants [3]. Studies in publication almost exclusively view gender through a binary lens, often using the terms sex and gender interchangeably. Thus, viewing research as patterns that can be borrowed from, considered, and explored—rather than prescribed—is an ethical and beneficial approach.

Facial Expression. Factors that influence communicators' facial expression include environment, emotional state, relationship of the communicators, context, and cultural factors, in addition to gender. Women have been found to engage in more exaggerated and frequently occurring facial expressions than men [7]. Women are more prone to engage in smiling behavior; however, smiling habits depend on age and external factors such as those noted above including environment and situation. In light of this pattern of smiling behavior, women are smiled at more than men. Therefore, the most frequent smiling interactions are found between woman-woman interactions, as opposed to man-man interactions where smiling patterns are found to be scarcer [8].

Eye Gaze. Eye contact and gaze patterns fall within the category of oculesics. Eye contact can be seen as a means to assert dominance, show interest, or convey attentive listening depending on the context in which the communication is taking place. Some patterns relating to eye contact and gaze vary between men and women in Western cultures. Women tend to engage in increased exploratory visual scanning as compared to men who maintain gaze at the eye region when looking at their communication partners [9]. Women also tend to make more eye contact and are gazed at more than men. Similar to smiling patterns, woman-woman interactions have the largest amount of eye contact [10]. Eye gaze behavior and meaning vary drastically from culture to culture. Where eye contact may be seen as a form of respect within one culture, it may be considered rude or even hostile in another. Eye contact can have a negative impact for folks who are neurodivergent. Individuals with self-declared autism spectrum disorder can experience adverse emotional and physiological reactions in addition to sensory overload while making eye contact [11].

Proxemics. Many factors influence the proximity of those involved in a given communication attempt [12]. Broadly, men tend to place distance between those they communicate with, while women tend to position themselves closer to communication partners. People in general tend to position themselves closer to women than men. Woman-woman interactions tend to have the closest proximity [10]. The spatial relationship between speaker and others for social interactions (interpersonal-comfort space) adjusts in response to threatening or unappealing facial expressions or the perception thereof [13, 14]. Culturally, research shows personal space shrinks or expands due to context differences between high-contact cultures and low-contact cultures [15].

Kinetics. In regard to kinetics and posture, the physical behavior of men has been observed to be more restless (fidgeting and foot/leg movements, tapping) as well as relaxed (leaning and feet on table) than women's physical behavior [10, 16]. Men tend to take up more physical space with wide leg and arm positioning, whereas women maintain a more contained resting position, depending on cultural and external factors. Women also tend to demonstrate more engaged listening body positioning through nodding and leaning forward toward their communication partners [3]. Women have been found to engage in more expressive body movements during speech through hand gestures, often mirroring the person with whom they are communicating, whereas men tend to have more static head movements [17].

Haptics. Though varying dramatically from culture to culture, context to context, and individual to individual, generally, in the USA women tend to engage in more self-touch than men, which is often perceived as a self-conscious, regulating behavior [10]. Women also are more likely to engage in casual touch with others during communication attempts, particularly with other women [18]. Hirsch and Boonin report that where women tend to use touch for expression and to convey warmth, men tend to use touch more as a means to demonstrate power, direct their communication partners, and express sexual interest [19].

Techniques to Facilitate Nonverbal Communication

Communication goes far beyond verbal communication and far beyond voice. The catalyst for SLP support with any aspects of nonverbal communication needs to come from the client. In an early conversation, the SLP can show how nonverbal behaviors are important to communication. Once the client acknowledges aspects they would like to modify, the SLP can create a safe space for exploring different choices for nonverbal communication.

SLPs may engage in meta-therapy to guide expectations about the process of modifying nonverbal aspects of communication [20]. An important dialogue that might occur is that intrinsic to the process of training nonverbal communication, attention is drawn to the body and the role it plays in expression and perception of gender. Discussing nonverbal communication may be sensitive, and putting attention on the body may be uncomfortable for individuals who have experiences of dysphoria, dysmorphia, or trauma. SLPs must gauge client comfort and discomfort that may arise. As needed, SLPs will need to adjust their support to promote a better context for exploring nonverbal communication.

Clients will need a safe place where they can freely practice their movement and expression. SLPs might include a dialogue around finding space to practice outside of sessions. By engaging in meta-therapy, the client can offer ideas for how they will arrive at or create a practice space. Within this, there may be varied comfort levels depending on the scenario, feeling in control and safe in certain social settings versus feeling uncomfortable with people less familiar.

Identifying skills in social competence is valuable to supporting nonverbal communication. By considering social competence throughout the process, movement and expression are grounded in intentional communication. Social competence skills include pragmatics, requesting attention, providing information, and sociorelational skills such as demonstrating interest or projecting a positive self-image. Supporting clients with nonverbal behaviors must tie movements and facial expressions to intentional communication acts in personally and professionally relevant scenarios and situations.

Visual perception plays a crucial role in training nonverbal communication behaviors. Analysis of others' nonverbal communication can be instructive [21]. The SLP may offer myriad gender representations of nonverbal communication by exposing clients to communicators of diverse genders who use a range of nonverbal behaviors. Becoming aware of the diversity of nonverbal communication styles can occur by reviewing recorded video footage of others as well as through live observation of people's actions, for example, in a park or at a restaurant. Clients may hone communication choices through watching these different communicators and noting their facial expressions, eye gaze, physical appearance, physical movements, proximity to others, and additional aspects of nonverbal communication. If comfortable, clients can build awareness of their current nonverbal behaviors by reviewing photographs and videos of themselves or observing themselves in a mirror. As their nonverbal behaviors change, clients can gain visual feedback with repeated photography or videography of themselves.

Movements and facial expressions communicate meaning or intention in our interactions. Creative movement and imitation are two approaches to developing different body movement patterns and facial expressions. In creative movement activities, clients use their body to make novel, unique movements and explore movement patterns through their environment. For example, a client can discover gait differences by walking with different parts of the body leading (e.g., forehead versus left hip). Creative opportunities bring awareness to the body, are channels for expression, and illustrate the interpersonal aspect of movements. In imitation, clients move as they see someone else move or "mirror" without verbalization. Clients replicate what they observe in others with their own face and body. SLPs should be mindful of clients with an array of physical abilities and varying rapport with their body. SLPs who apply movement-based training should center clients in deciding how to move and obtain consent for any tactile approaches.

Training of movements and facial expressions may consider principles of motor learning. In this learning approach, the SLP can provide instructions that attach the movement pattern or facial expression to an effect such as communicative intent. For example, clinicians may provide the instruction to make a movement signaling the desire to speak or make a facial expression conveying interest in what someone is saying. The SLP can provide variable practice by providing different scenarios in which the nonverbal communication could occur. For example, the client can show how they would signal the desire to speak at work versus at home as well as with a supervisor versus a co-worker. SLPs should avoid providing biomechanical instructions on how clients should position themselves or make a facial expression. Instead of commenting on the body position, the SLP can provide an observation that the movement did or did not convey a certain communicative intent.

Role-play is useful in training nonverbal communication behaviors. The SLP proposes a communication situation, and the client identifies learned nonverbal behaviors. The client also describes how different circumstances impact their nonverbal communication behaviors. With this knowledge, the SLP encourages the client to explore moving in different ways in response to a situation. The SLP guides the client in contrastive practice, a technique requiring clients to demonstrate their current behavior and a new behavior. By juxtaposing current and novel behaviors, the client gains awareness and control of physical behaviors that contribute to their nonverbal communication. In line with a trauma-informed approach, SLPs should gain clear consent prior to demonstrating techniques through tactile approaches.

Changing communication behaviors can be difficult. Mindfulness is a useful approach to bring awareness to our emotional state and the physiologic reactions that accompany them. While mindfulness often directs a client's focus inward toward internal sensations, mindfulness can bring awareness to external circumstances. The SLP can engage the client in a mindfulness activity in which they sit quietly in a room where other people are interacting. The client silently observes the environment they are in as well as others' nonverbal behaviors, watching without judgment. After a period of observation, the client reflects on any nonverbal aspects.

Through this activity, the SLP can learn and explore nonverbal behaviors that appeal to the client.

Another reflective practice is journaling. Whether written, typed, or audio-recorded, the journal provides a location to collate information that represents their unique experience. With journaling, clients accumulate a collection of thoughts that they can revisit. Clients may describe their perspective on specific communication situations or note others' reactions to them. Similarly, clients can create a vision board where they amass images that represent their desired expression. Together, these metacognitive activities provide clients the opportunity to consider their goals for nonverbal communication and convey their feelings about the process.

The need for counseling can surface when exploring new communication behaviors. Exploring nonverbal communication behaviors, in particular, may evoke strong emotional reactions that require skills in counseling. While the SLP is not a counselor or psychologist, the SLP has training and skills to deal with obstacles that limit progress in communication goals. For example, changes in comfortability may occur with one's transition and others adjusting to it. A counseling point to the client could be that they can adjust their proxemics in any situation to signal their boundaries because the comfortable distance between communicators is negotiable [14].

Generalization to Communication Situations

The ultimate goal for any training process is transferring what is learned in sessions to everyday communication situations. Allowing the client to lead that aspect of the training process is critical. If a client's goal is to develop nonverbal behaviors they perceive as more "feminine" or "androgynous," a client may identify which of their nonverbal communication behaviors they consider "masculine" and in what scenarios or social environments they feel they still need to use those behaviors to feel accepted. A client can recognize spaces that are safe to let those behaviors go and try new ones, deciding which traits to keep and which to modify [14, 22]. As clients increase their self-efficacy in their nonverbal communication, clients decide which situations and contexts they have as safe options to integrate nonverbal aspects that support their expression of self.

Pitfalls and Considerations

- **Clinician personal biases.** Every clinician inevitably brings their own set of personal biases, particularly on a topic as ingrained as gender perception and expression. Clinicians must acknowledge and unpack these biases prior to working with transgender and gender nonconforming individuals. Exploration of personal biases around gender can take place individually, although any clinician wanting to practice in this area should attend transgender-led training on cultural responsiveness and gender-affirming language.

- **Client commitment.** A component that impacts progress and satisfaction that is less within a clinician's control is client commitment. Client commitment can be variable throughout the process depending on a number of factors including discomfort with attention to the body [23]. If client commitment seems to be fading, the appropriate course of action is checking in with clients to determine the reason(s) for change in follow-through. The clinician supports the client's lead on whether or not to continue adapting throughout the therapy process to clients' evolving goals.
- **Evolving terminology.** Rhetoric is continuously shifting and evolving, which is especially true for the transgender, gender nonconforming, and gender-diverse community that has historically been marginalized with rhetoric shifted and weaponized against them to cause harm. As a means to be more inclusive, reduce harm, promote expression, and follow a natural progression of language adaptation, terminology used by this population to describe themselves is ever-evolving. For example, terms in the vernacular 10 years ago may carry offensive connotations today. While asking clients what terms they use to refer to themselves is advisable, it is not ethical to rely on clients to keep you updated with current appropriate terminology. It is part of the clinician's duty to stay up to date on current language and research.
- **Being prescriptive.** Limiting possibilities to the binary view of female or male and masculine or feminine is highly problematic. Gender is a spectrum, and interpretation and expression of gender are deeply personal and can be fluid. Existing research into perception of nonverbal communication aspects using predominantly cisgender participants should not be used as a layout for therapy, but rather something that clients can explore when modifying behavior. Clients can borrow components that resonate with them and leave aspects that do not. When sharing research, it is important to preface with a statement that current literature provides an exceedingly limited, binary, and often outdated viewpoint. Instead of a prescriptive, binary approach, the SLP can offer a compassionate, explorative viewpoint recognizing that gender varies greatly from person to person. Therapy success is based on client satisfaction when the client feels they have achieved their goals. The SLP's role is to guide and support clients' goals, allowing for shifting and fluidity throughout the process.

References

1. Purnell L. Cross cultural communication: verbal and non-verbal communication, interpretation and translation. In: Douglas M, Pacquiao D, Purnell L, editors. Global applications of culturally competent health care: guidelines for practice. Cham: Springer; 2018.
2. Payrató L. Non-verbal communication. In: Verschueren J, Ostman JO, editors. Key notions for pragmatics. Amsterdam: John Benjamins Publishing Company; 2009.

3. Hardy TLD, Boliek CA, Aalto D, Lewicke J, Wells K, Rieger JM. Contributions of voice and nonverbal communication to perceived masculinity-femininity for cisgender and transgender communicators. J Speech Lang Hear Res. 2020;63(4):931–47. https://doi.org/10.1044/2019_JSLHR-19-00387.
4. Van Borsel J, De Cuypere G, Van den Berghe H. Physical appearance and voice in male-to-female transsexuals. J Voice. 2001;15(4):570–5. https://doi.org/10.1016/S0892-1997(01)00059-5.
5. Van Borsel J, de Pot K, De Cuypere G. Voice and physical appearance in female-to-male transsexuals. J Voice. 2009;23(4):494–7.
6. American Speech-Language-Hearing Association. Scope of practice in speech-language pathology [Scope of Practice]. 2016. www.asha.org/policy/.
7. Kring AM, Gordon AH. Sex differences in emotion: expression, experience, and physiology. J Pers Soc Psychol. 1998;74:686–703.
8. LaFrance M, Hecht MA, Levy Paluck E. The contingent smile: a meta-analysis of sex differences in smiling. Psychol Bull. 2003;129:305–34.
9. Coutrot A, Binetti N, Harrison C, Mareschal I, Johnston A. Gaze behavior provides a gender fingerprint. J Vision (Charlottesville Va.). 2016;16(12):71. https://doi.org/10.1167/16.12.71.
10. Hall JA. Nonverbal gender differences: communication accuracy and expressive style. Baltimore, MD: The Johns Hopkins University Press; 1984.
11. Trevisan DA, Roberts N, Lin C, Birmingham E. How do adults and teens with self-declared autism spectrum disorder experience eye contact? A qualitative analysis of first-hand accounts. PLoS One. 2017;12(11):e0188446. https://doi.org/10.1371/journal.pone.0188446.
12. Albas C. Proxemic behavior: a study of extrusion. J Psychol. 1991;131(5):697–702.
13. Ruggiero G, Rapuanol M, Cartaud A, Coello Y, Iachini T. Defensive functions provoke similar psychophysiological reactions in reaching and comfort spaces. Sci Rep. 2021;11:5170. https://doi.org/10.1038/s41598-021-83988-2.
14. McCall C, Singer T. Facing off with unfair others: introducing proxemic imaging as an implicit measure of approach and avoidance during social interaction. PLoS One. 2015;10(2):e0117532. https://doi.org/10.1371/journal.pone.0117532.
15. Høgh-Olesen H. Human spatial behaviour: the spacing of people, objects and animals in six cross-cultural samples. J Cogn Cult. 2008;8(2008):245–80. https://doi.org/10.1163/156853708X358173.
16. Glass L. He says, she says: closing the communication gap between sexes. New York, NY: G.P. Putnam and Sons; 1992.
17. Nelson A, Golant SK. You don't say: navigating nonverbal communication between the sexes. New York, NY: Prentice-Hall; 2004.
18. Hall JA. Gender and status patterns in social touch. In: Hertenstein M, editor. The handbook of touch: neuroscience, behavioral, and health perspectives. New York: Springer; 2011. p. 329–50.
19. Hirsch S, Boonin J. Nonverbal communication: assessment and training considerations across the gender and cultural spectrum. In: Adler R, Hirsch S, Pickering J, editors. Voice and communication therapy for the transgender/gender diverse client: a comprehensive clinical guide. 3rd ed. San Diego, CA: Plural Publishing; 2019. p. 249–80.
20. Helou LB, Gartner-Schmidt JL, Hapner ER, Schneider SL, Van Stan JH. Mapping meta-therapy in voice interventions onto the rehabilitation treatment specification system. Semin Speech Lang. 2021;42(01):5–18.
21. Gilchrist JD, Solomon-Krakus S, Pila E, Crocker P, Sabiston CM. Associations between physical self-concept and anticipated guilt and shame: the moderating role of gender. Sex Roles. 2020;83:763–72. https://doi.org/10.1007/s11199-020-01137-x.
22. Worthington RL, Reynolds AL. Within-group differences in sexual orientation and identity. J Couns Psychol. 2009;56(1):44–55. https://doi.org/10.1037/a0013498.
23. Lin C-S, Ku H-L, Chao H-T, Tu P-C, Li C-T, et al. Neural network of body representation differs between transsexuals and cissexuals. PLoS One. 2014;9(1):e85914. https://doi.org/10.1371/journal.pone.0085914.

Chapter 10
The Singing Voice

Felix A. Graham

Introduction

Vocal training of the transgender and gender non-conforming (TGNC) individuals presents a myriad of conditional challenges as each singer's vocal journey is unique to their personal circumstances. Singing offers unparalleled opportunities for self-expression and development of self-identity. While it is particularly helpful to individuals who are considering or pursuing gender transition, there are barriers to entry, often in the form of incongruence between voice and gender identities, as well as limited access to appropriate or identity-sensitive vocal instruction. This chapter seeks to give voice practitioners insight into appropriate modalities for gender-affirming singing voice training, as well as a broad survey of the potential challenges and interventions related to the TGNC community. Observations from clinical practice and evidence-based vocal and pedagogical tools are offered as a guide to balancing healthy, sustainable phonation with the singer's transitional goals.

The overall structure and approach to training for TGNC voices is similar to other singing populations, in that decisions must be made around the individual's unique voice and situation. Regardless of a client's gender identity, individualized approaches based in the principles of voice production, learner-centric pedagogy, and collaborative music-making—the voice professional's toolbox—still apply.

F. A. Graham (✉)
Independent Scholar, New York, NY, USA
e-mail: felix@singwithdrfelix.com

M. S. Courey et al. (eds.), *Voice and Communication in Transgender and Gender Diverse Individuals*, https://doi.org/10.1007/978-3-031-24632-6_10

Techniques derived from current pedagogical research, when thoughtfully applied, can expand current vocal training practices toward a more gender-inclusive model, help transgender voice clients feel more at ease in the vocal studio, and significantly aid their progress.

Background

While rudimentary laryngoscopy techniques were developed in the early nineteenth century, with voice treatments growing increasingly more sophisticated since then [1], the intricate nature of the vocal mechanism still limits the types of direct interventions made available to transgender-identified singers. Accordingly, transgender-identified singers *assigned male at birth* (AMAB) are primarily limited to functional interventions—using scientifically informed pedagogical practices to shift the singer's vocal technique toward a lighter mechanism, with a higher brighter sound commonly associated with singers assigned female at birth (AFAB).

Of course, scientifically informed vocal training is not a new practice: Treatises on technique, as well as the physiology and function of singing, exist from the seventeent and eighteenth centuries. Voice professionals then, as now, exhibited curiosity in understanding the vocal mechanism and modifying their approaches based on their scientific understanding [2, 3]. Traditionally, however, vocal pedagogy has been sharply defined by the gender binary, with little consideration given to individuals whose post-pubertal voice conflicts with their gender identity. Seventeenth- and eighteenth-century singers in the western tradition conjure images of the gender-ambiguous *castrati*—male singers whose voices never completed pubertal development, giving them an androgynous sound. Yet pedagogical texts from the period seem directed primarily to the unmodified adult male voice, ignoring women and castrati completely despite their prevalence in the performing sphere [2]. Miller further notes that female singers and castrati were, in the seventeenth and eighteenth centuries, known and celebrated in society, but (perhaps similarly to how the course of medical research has historically minimized women) vocal experts at the time likely approached technique with a one-gender-fits-all lens. Thus, in a climate where gender roles controlled access to musical careers, where female singers and even castrati were functionally invisible to the experts of the day, it is unsurprising that the terminology that developed around voice and singing had inherently gendered implications [4].

As the vocal community's desire to accommodate and welcome transgender-identified singers has grown, the historic legacy of a highly gendered pedagogical tradition has become increasingly apparent. At the time of this publication, it should be noted that there is an ongoing communal discussion concerning all aspects of vocal pedagogy through the lens of gender inclusivity. One particularly vigorous topic of debate concerns the use of traditional voice types. Labeling singers as soprano, alto, tenor, and bass may seem innocuous on the surface, yet there are gendered implications to those terms, potentially alienating transgender singers whose gender identities do not align with the label their voice has received [4, 5]. While some transgender-identified singers may have no intrinsic objection to the use of such labels, one cannot assume that such labels accurately encapsulate a client's gender identity or preferred vocal outcomes. There is a considerable variety in gender expression among cis-female and cis-male voices, and this remains true in the transgender population as well: Even strongly female-identified singers may choose to use their current vocal range, while non-binary singers may choose to train toward a more traditionally feminine sound.[1]

Currently, there is no singular answer that satisfies everyone concerning terminology, but describing voices in terms of *tessitura* (comfortable singing range), *timbre* (the color of the voice), principal *octave*, or even by muscle function (i.e., *cricothyroid-dominant* and *thyroarytenoid-dominant*) are examples of ways to discuss voice without applying gendered labels to the voice itself, a shift that could benefit cis-gender singers, too [7].

Further complicating the issue of training for TGNC singing voices is the lack of relevant literature. Much of the research on TGNC voice is either directed at medical or spoken voice interventions, and the body of literature concerning the TGNC singing voice primarily concerns the effects of HRT on singers *assigned female at birth* (AFAB). While Kozan and Hammond [8] directly address practical methods, the body of literature overwhelmingly focuses on social issues and cultural competency, rather than experimental or action research directly related to the training of transgender voices [8–13]. Accordingly, the techniques outlined in this chapter pull from existing knowledge from surrounding fields, as well as observations and experiences from transgender-identified singing voice specialists. Because the communal understanding of certain terms in vocal pedagogy may differ from person to person, a table of definitions is provided below to clarify usage and intent (Table 10.1).

[1] "Traditionally feminine" is, of course, relative to one's cultural background, communal norms, orientation, and age. The author recognizes that there are many ways, often conflicting, to talk about gender, voice, and transition. Even within transgender communities, there is an ongoing discourse around what constitutes sensitive language when discussing topics such as adolescent puberty, voice change, and gendered expectations, and literature recognizes the rapidly changing nature of language in the field of transgender studies [6]. The language choices here are reflective of the author's own experience as a transgender voice professional and will not always be generalizable to every situation. As in all things, when in doubt, the best practice is to approach every situation with flexibility and respect toward the client's stated preferences.

Table 10.1 Definitions of terminology as used in this chapter

Terms	Definition and usage
Aspiration, aspirated phonation	Phonation that is breathy, fuzzy, or airy, due to insufficient closure of the vocal folds. This may result from poor adduction due to muscle weakness or lack of coordination, purposeful breathiness, or muscle tension
Cricothyroid, CT	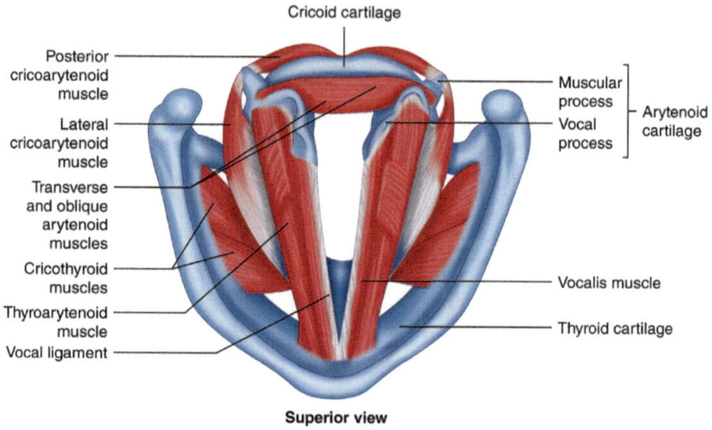 Intrinsic musculature of the larynx While *cricothyroid* on its own is a specific muscle set, in vocal pedagogy the terms are commonly used to refer to the entire collection of intrinsic muscles of the larynx that directly or indirectly control closure and thinning of the folds (affecting pitch and registration). See the above **figure** for reference
CT-dominant	Phonation wherein the cricothyroid muscle set predominantly controls the shifts to the vocal mechanism during singing. Head voice, falsetto (or "flipped voice"), whistle, and even mixed voice can be referred to as CT-dominant. CT-dominance is also associated with vocal efficiency, "top-down" phonation. While CT-dominant function is more commonly associated with AFAB voices, there are many AMAB voices that are predominantly CT-dominant
Embouchure	The shape of the mouth (usually in reference to vowel formation) while phonating. Spreading, or a wide embouchure, raises the larynx, while a closed embouchure tends to encourage a lower laryngeal posture
Flipped voice	Sudden change from the lower vocal register (usually a chest voice or TA-dominant sound) to a higher vocal register (head voice or falsetto). "Flipped voice" is used as a gender-neutral way to refer to what has traditionally been referred to as falsetto in AMAB voices
Glottal, glottal attacks, hard glottal attack	A hard, sudden closure of the vocal folds that results in a loud, abrupt phonatory onset. Hard glottal attacks are often a sign of either muscular tension, anxiety about pitch, or phonation in general—Often both at the same time. Frequent hard glottal attacks can be a source of phonotrauma, i.e., damage to the vocal fold tissue

Table 10.1 (continued)

Terms	Definition and usage
Habilitative, habilitation	Habilitative vocal training is the prevention of vocal damage through the training (or retraining) of healthy phonation habits and technique. This is in contrast to *rehabilitation*, which is the reversal of physiological injury or dysfunction. While habilitative training may indirectly correct injury or dysfunction, rehabilitation is not the primary purpose of the training. Therapists *rehabilitate*; voice teachers and singing specialists *habilitate*
Head voice, chest voice, mix voice	Labels which are frequently used to talk about *registration*—The modes in which the vocal mechanism shifts when moving from one end of the pitch range to the other. Recent trends tend to use terms such as *modes*, *CT-dominance/TA-dominance*, or even *heavy* vs. *light* mechanism, as the terms head, chest, and mix can be confusing in context and do not always accurately convey the changes in mechanism that need to occur. In this chapter, head voice is associated with CT-dominance and light mechanism, whereas chest is associated with TA-dominance and heavy mechanism. Mix voice is a blend between the two which can have varying degrees of lightness and heaviness
Onset	The manner in which the muscles of the larynx bring the vocal folds together (*adduction*) to begin the sound. Onset is an essential part of healthy phonation and exists on a spectrum from *hard glottal attack* to *soft aspirated attack.* Efficient onsets fall somewhere in the middle of the spectrum
Phonotrauma	Onsets, phonation, or tension (sometimes all three at once) that cause micro-trauma to the vocal folds. This can include singing or speaking habits, as well as other kinds of phonatory behavior, such as coughing, clearing the throat, etc.
Pressed phonation	Singing or speaking where the vocalist uses the extrinsic musculature of the vocal mechanism, such as the constrictors or glossus (tongue), to "squeeze" the vocal folds together. This often occurs as a response to aspirated sounds, used in an attempt to create a clearer sound. This type of phonation can lead to fatigue, injury, or even compensatory dysfunction
Registration, register breaks, passaggio	Registration refers to the four distinct types of phonatory patterns observed in the human voice. "Register" encompasses multiple factors, such as muscle dominance, laryngeal posturing, tone color (*timbre*), and pitch. Traditionally, these have been labeled in terms such as *fry*, *chest*, *head*, *falsetto*, or *whistle.* Breaks or *passaggio* points are the range of pitches wherein the change from one register to another is audible
Semi-occluded vocal tract (SOVT)	SOVT refers to the practice of *occluding*—That is, partially blocking—The mouth to build up pressure in the mouth, above the vocal folds. This has the effect of stabilizing the larynx, as it equalizes the air pressure above the folds with the air pressure below the folds (see *subglottal pressure* below). This has many potential benefits, such as training the singer to use less air pressure, reduce collision (impact of the vocal folds coming together), release tension, and find a more resonant sound
Subglottal pressure, pressurization	Subglottal pressure refers to the air pressure beneath the vocal folds during phonation. Excess pressure can create tension and vocal dysfunction, prevent appropriate shifts in registration, and limit vocal range. AMAB voices tend to use more subglottal pressure than AFAB voices, which can cause phonotrauma or inhibit the progress of vocal transition if left unaddressed

(continued)

Table 10.1 (continued)

Terms	Definition and usage
Tessitura	The range of pitches wherein voice function is most efficient. Voice labels often are references to the range in which a voice can comfortably sing for a period of time. This is separate from *range*, which is simply the spread of pitches a voice can sing
Thin-edge phonation	The lip of the vocal fold (where the two folds touch) shifts in thickness as pitch is raised and lowered. The fold must be naturally thin as the voice ascends in pitch, and the thin lip or edge occurs when going into the higher modes of the voice (particularly in *flipped* or falsetto modes). Thin-edge phonation refers to the practice of bringing the sensation of that lightness and thinness down into the lower range, where the folds naturally thicken. When the sensation of the thin edge is brought down into the lower voice, it can assist in creating the lighter, brighter sound that is associated with AFAB voices
Thyroarytenoid, TA	The thyroarytenoid muscles refer to the vocal folds themselves (see above figure). The *CT* muscles work antagonistically to the TA, stretching and thinning the muscles to allow the voice to ascend in pitch
TA-dominant	Phonation wherein the thyroarytenoids are the predominant source of muscle control. This is often referred to as chest voice, modal voice, or mode 1. While TA-dominant function is more commonly associated with AMAB voices, there are many AFAB voices that are predominantly TA-dominant

Singing and the Singer: A Holistic Approach to Vocal Training

Initial Sessions

Rapport-Building

While discussion of vocal training has traditionally offered technical advice and practical exercises for the singer (both of which will also be addressed later in this chapter), current pedagogical trends shift focus toward a holistic approach to voice training, which acknowledges the role of social interaction in successful voice training. Trust is fundamental to any effective teacher-student interactions, but building a secure teacher-student relationship is particularly crucial when working with the TGNC population [14]. Establishing a sense of social comfort with a student begins long before any actual singing tasks have been undertaken, and simple missteps in initial communication around social norms and appropriate vocabulary can have an immense impact on potential clients. Broader issues of cultural competency are addressed elsewhere in this text and thus will not be revisited; equally important in establishing a secure, inclusive learning environment, however, is building teacher-student *rapport* [15–17].

The necessity of rapport, long established in the literature as an important component of musical learning, intensifies when issues of voice and identity are at stake. Singing for assessment with a new teacher or coach is anxiety-inducing under the best circumstances, and if the singer is concerned about how their gender identity will be perceived and received, that anxiety is understandably amplified [13, 18]. As vocal assessment is intrinsically hindered without understanding the client's goals, the voice professional should give considerable attention toward understanding their identity, transition journey, and vocal goals prior to vocalization. Traditional practice has been to immediately vocalize new clients to hear the voice and determine which interventions may be needed. Yet, rushing into vocalization or insisting the client demonstrate uncomfortable areas of the voice may inhibit the rapport-building process. Until confidence in the voice professional's readiness to hear and address vocal needs is established and mutual trust is built, incremental steps forward guided by the client's comfort level is recommended.

Consultation/Vocal Counseling

An initial intake process for new or potential clients is recommended; it is important to understand a client's desires prior to any vocal work. For TGNC singers, this is imperative, as the voice professional cannot suggest interventions without understanding both the client's level of vocal understanding and desired outcomes. An initial counseling session allows the voice professional to gain insight into the singer's background, their vocal history, their goals and aspirations, as well as offering a chance to build rapport with the singer prior to vocalization [19, 20]. There are many vocal assessment methods and forms, ranging from the medically focused to artistic assessment, and each practitioner will develop their own approach. A sample procedure, which is adapted from Titze and Verdolini Abbott [20], is found in Appendix 1 and may be used as a broad guide toward developing an assessment method for individual practice.

The shape of the initial counseling session shifts according to the knowledge and singing level of the client: Those with professional aspirations and experience will likely already have some understanding of voice and the limitations of physiology, while new or avocational singers may lack the knowledge or experience to determine what outcomes are possible for their instrument. In the former case, the counseling session will allow the voice professional to understand the singer's technical background and determine what interventions have already been tried; in the latter, there may need to be gentle but frank discussion around expectations and potential outcomes. Establishing an emphasis on healthy, efficient vocalization within the bounds of the individual's unique physiology from the outset can help address unrealistic expectations or single-minded focus on a specific outcome while maintaining the singer's motivation, confidence, and enthusiasm.

Expectations and Outcomes: Emphasizing Function over Sound

A primary challenge of voice training for transfeminine and AMAB non-binary singers lies in the limitation of medical interventions for voice feminization. Feminizing HRT, begun after adolescent voice change, has a negligible impact on the physiological vocal mechanism.[2] Potential TGNC voice outcomes and interventions are not yet widely understood, and clients may approach vocal training with unrealistic expectations. Even outcomes that are achievable for some may be out of reach for others, simply due to their unique circumstances. This knowledge gap creates situations where singers may focus on comparisons to others and judge themselves based on outcomes, rather than their own relative progress. This friction around outcomes, internal satisfaction, and identity may be minimized or avoided altogether by structuring counseling and training around function, rather than sound. Shifting the singer's focus toward function can be achieved by addressing voice transition from two directions: *social* vocal transition vs. *technical* vocal transition.

Social Vocal Transition

Social focus begins in the initial sessions by determining how the client envisions using their voice, rather than how the voice sounds. *Authenticity*, *freedom*, *expressiveness*, *creativity*, and ease of *communication* are useful terms to shape this inquiry, and these are topics worth revisiting from time to time as clients may not readily have answers and need time and space to consider. Focus on social function builds the singer's sense of personal agency, using objective measures of progress ("Am I using my voice in a way that makes me feel confident in myself?") rather than subjective measures ("Do I sound ____ enough?"). Further, when a singer can see measurable progress, their intrinsic motivation to practice and challenge themselves is encouraged. This is invaluable for TGNC clients, as stimulating intrinsic motivation and self-efficacy is a necessary component of perceived competency, lowered performance anxiety, and personal satisfaction in one's voice [21–25].

Technical Vocal Transition

Technique and mechanical training should also focus on process, physiological feedback, and vocal exploration, rather than specific outcomes. This begins with assessing vocal function: Is the singer able to vocalize freely throughout their range? Is there balanced registration, energetic breath flow, and appropriate pressurization during phonation? *Semi-occluded vocal tract* (SOVT) exercises such as straw phonation, glides on a closed /u/, or voiced fricatives are useful for immediate assessment of function [20, 26]. As the vocalization progresses, the client should be asked to describe the sensations they experience; in cases where singers may not have the vocabulary or experience to respond, the following techniques may be useful:

(a) *Comparison*—The singer compares two different components, such as pitches, intervals, vowels, or types of exercises, e.g., "Which feels easier, the first vowel or the second?"

[2] This is not to say that HRT has no potential effect on the vocal function, however. There are considerations relevant to the singing voice, addressed later on in this chapter.

(b) *Spectrum*—The singer ranks vocalizations or iterations of exercises on a spectrum, such as *free or easy* vs. *restricted or tight* or *relaxed* vs. *tense*.
(c) *Experiential*—The singer describes the experience of vocalization in a metaphorical way, such as the emotional or visualized experience while phonating.

Exercises should be described to client in terms of how they address the physiological function of the voice and the desired outcome, and the description need not be technically complex. A simple cause-and-effect description often suffices: "Try singing through a straw to relax the throat; that may help you reach this note more easily." Function should remain the primary focus even when assessing repertoire or sound production, and one should consistently seek feedback from the client about their sensory experience of singing. Even if produced sound matches the desired outcome, the client may experience functional tension, and verbally reinforcing the importance of the sound over efficiency may result in vocal manipulations that are ultimately harmful.

This dualistic approach to vocal instruction draws from many fields of pedagogical practice, including constructivist, cognitive, and motor learning theories [20, 27, 28]. Teaching conscious awareness and attention as well as deliberate practice rather than mechanical rehearsal requires an initial time investment that may seem costly at the outset. However, the benefits—modeling efficient solo practice, increased self-awareness, improved teacher-student communication, and decreased performance anxiety—are numerous and well-documented in pedagogical literature [29–31].

Paths to Technical Vocal Transition

The underlying principle of vocal feminization lies in the adjustment of resonance, registration, and vocal function to create the lighter, brighter sound associated with cis-female vocalization. Though fundamental phonatory frequency is sometimes seen as the primary cue for vocal gender identification, research suggests that voice identification takes many different aspects into account—pitch, yes, but also resonance or timbre, diction, and situationally specific use. This suggests that one or more vocal characteristics, such as pitch, may be gender atypical so long as other aspects align with social expectations of femininity [32–35].

This, however, presumes that the client wishes to be perceived as cis-female, which may not be the case. Here, different approaches to vocal transition are offered that take client preference into account. For singers training the voice after adolescent voice change, there are three general paths of singing voice transition: *unmodified*, where the client maintains their post-pubertal vocal registration, range, and timbre; *hybrid*, where the client may choose to make certain alterations, such as timbral shifts, but maintain the core range and method of vocal production; and *modified*, where the client shifts registration, range, and timbre entirely. The choice of approach will be dictated primarily by the client's transition goals and individual voice, though age, prior experience, and frequency of practice will affect potential outcomes.

The Unmodified Voice

Some clients may choose to undergo no appreciable shift to their singing voice for many reasons. Some may wish to maintain the instrument for professional reasons, while others may see their voice as an artifact or record of their life and have no desire to change it. In these cases, range, registration breaks, and tuning strategies will take a similar path to their male cis-gender counterparts. Whether or not the client uses traditional labels (tenor, baritone, bass) is an individual choice, and the best practice is using neutral terms (e.g., flipped, high, middle, or low voice) where practicable. Clients pursuing HRT may require technical adjustments to accommodate any resulting shifts in vocal function. This may include reducing fold impact, particularly at higher frequencies; improving vocal efficiency through resonant voice strategies to decrease strain; softening onsets; and optimizing both airflow and subglottal pressurization. Suggested approaches include SOVT techniques, focus on both upper- and lower-body expansions to reduce air pressure, and exercises designed for flexibility of the vocal folds.

The Hybrid Voice

Other clients may choose to make some vocal adjustments, such as shifts to a brighter resonance and lighter phonatory mechanism, while still maintaining the core instrument's tessitura, singing range, and technical approach. Some voice professionals' experience suggests that this is often the path that non-binary singers choose as it gives them options for expressing themselves with both masculine- and feminine-coded vocal timbres. Here, again, neutral voice labels are useful. In these cases, interventions focus on strengthening *cricothyroid* (CT) function, modifying airflow (*support*) to accommodate a lighter phonation (*head voice* or *mix*) with a higher laryngeal position for brighter resonance where desired. Top-down vocal function exercises and *yodeling* (deliberate register shifts) will aid in building that mix and reducing register entanglement; this is key to maintaining the lighter mix without fatigue. It should be noted in general that developing CT function is beneficial to singers of all voice types and genres to maintain the health of the instrument. Suggested approaches include guiding the singer toward self-monitoring of laryngeal posture and consciously resetting the laryngeal position during inhalation when necessary, as well as using SOVT techniques in the middle and upper register to drop excessive weight and prevent over-pressurization as they ascend in pitch.

The Modified Voice

This final category includes clients who may wish to train their voices to a phonatory style associated with cis-female singers. Labels such as *countertenor* or *falsettist* should be avoided altogether; alto or soprano may be useful to describe the approach to the client, but the client should lead in applying those labels to themselves. Using the term *flipped voice* rather than falsetto helps reinforce the idea that function is gender-neutral, rather than associated with binary sex.

For this transition path, there must be a balance between building and strengthening both CT-dominant function via top-down phonatory exercises and maintaining healthy function of the thyroarytenoid-dominant (TA) register. Clients may be reluctant to use their modal range because of gender incongruity in the sound, but reframing exercises in this area as functional work, rather than sound, often resolves this friction. Exercises that focus on *thin-edge* phonation with an open throat but small, rounded embouchure are useful for clients who have difficulty accessing their upper range.[3] Suggested approaches include exercises to work on fold thinning with controlled airflow, such as top-down /vi/ sirens, staccati on /u/, and yodeling from a heavy lower sound to a light upper voice.

Beginning singers may have an advantage in this approach, as they are not bringing phonatory muscle memory of heavier registration into their singing. In all cases, however, clients must understand that even though there are immediate gains to be made, this approach takes significant time and consistent, regular practice. Small chunks of focused practice two or three times a day may be more efficacious than long sessions, particularly if the client experiences vocal fatigue when singing for longer periods of time.

Sample Exercises (Table 10.2)

The exercises included here are suitable for all three approaches detailed above—when, where, and how to use them will be dependent on the singer, the goals, and even the status or condition of the voice from day to day. For efficiency, exercises should address more than one function, in no small part because every function of the vocal mechanism is influenced to some degree by the others: Breath affects registration, which affects resonance, which in turn hinders or helps articulation, for example. References to yodeling or flipped voice in these exercises refer to the dramatic shift from the lowest (chest) register to the highest flipped (falsetto) register (Fig. 10.1).

Table 10.2 IPA legend for sample exercises

Vowel sounds used in the exercise examples
o as in CODE
ɔ as in CAUGHT
eɪ as in MAY
e as in SHAVE
i as in FEET
ɑ as in FATHER
æ as in CAT
ɛ as in MET
u as in TOO

[3] This approach is sometimes referred to as *cuperto* in traditional, classical vocal technique.

a **Easy, narrow onset, thin-edge fold and light phonation**

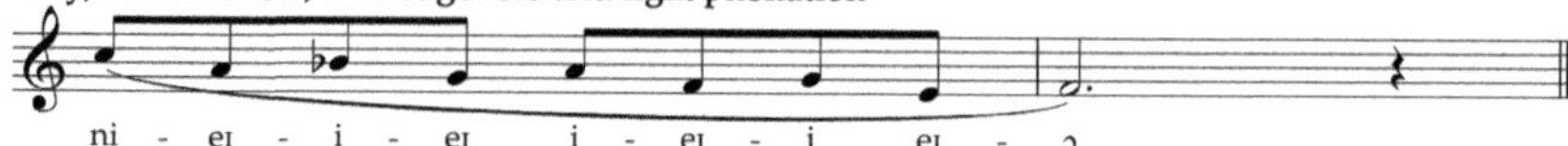

Begin in singer's comfortable flipped range and come down to the low voice, using the 'n' to start the sound with a narrow focus and 'i' for the thin-edge fold. Keep the 'eɪ' and the 'ɔ' in the same narrow groove created by the 'ni', and focus on keeping the sound lifted all the way down. The last note should not drop, shift registers heavily or change color significantly. The final vowel may shift the teach the voice to bring the narrowness, height and lightness into all of the heavier vowels, such as 'ɛ' or 'ɑ'.

Flexibility, lightening the voice, straw phonation

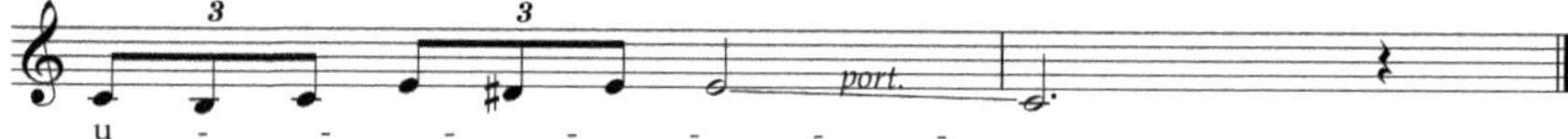

Have the singer sing an 'u' into a straw, with the embouchure rounded around the straw stem. Depending on the singer's level and comfort in higher voice, you may begin lower and work up, or higher and work down. Lightness should kept throughout and brought down to the bottom note. The singer should keep the triplets as legato as possible and focus on keeping the throat open and tongue relaxed. The feeling of the open throat can be approximated by inhaling through the straw.

b **Reducing vocal fold impact**

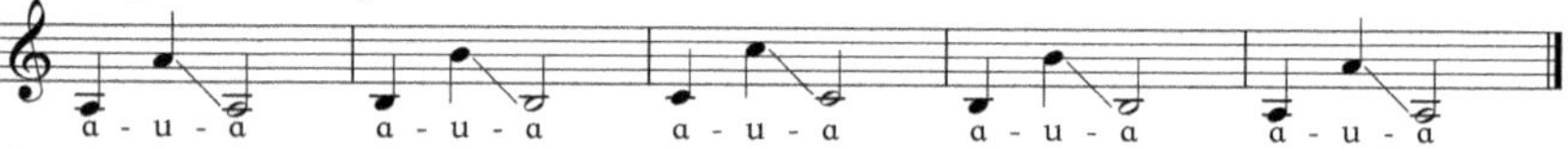

Begin in singer's low range, yodel (flip) up to the top note, then gently portamento down, maintaining lightness. This can be taken up through head voice into flipped voice, but should always come back down to bring the laryngeal position back into a relaxed posture. If the voice struggles with heaviness on the top, or has difficulty with the yodel, use æ instead of ɑ on the lower note to encourage the flip. Make sure the lips are clearly rounded and almost closed on the u.

Thin-edge phonation, easy onset, pressure reduction

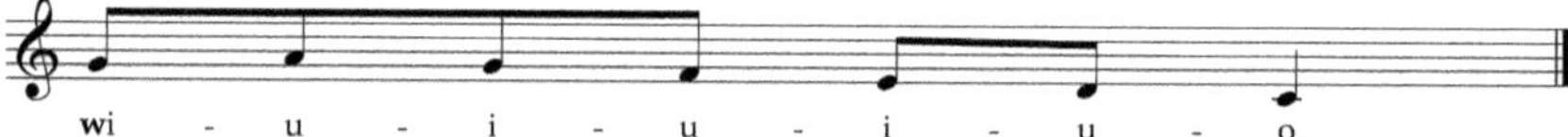

Begin in singer's comfortable falsetto range, emphasizing the glide (w) to bring the vocal folds together gently. Visualize the sound as being a thin, narrow ribbon or stream, and bring the feeling of lightness and narrowness down through the head voice / mix, into chest, never letting the placement drop.

c **Flexibility, lightening the voice, *cuperto* exercise**

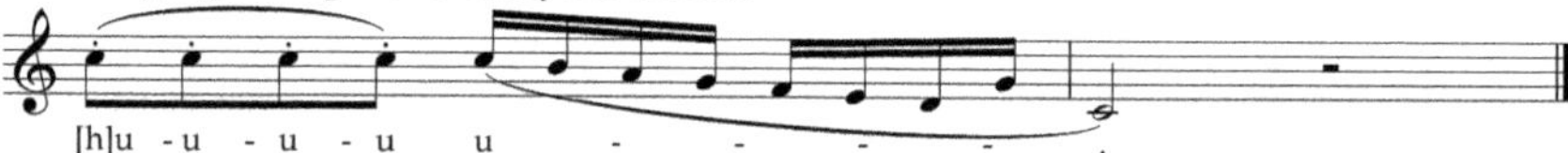

Depending on the singer's level and comfort in higher voice, you may begin lower and work up, or higher and work down. Lightness should kept throughout and brought down to the bottom note. The h at the beginning should only be used in the early stages to help the singer feel the gentleness of the onset. After that, the h should be *imagined*, rather than sung. The throat should be open, while the mouth is rounded into a small 'u' shape with the tongue relaxed. The feeling of the open throat can be approximated by inhaling through the small embouchure.

Yodel for dropping weight and reducing register entanglement

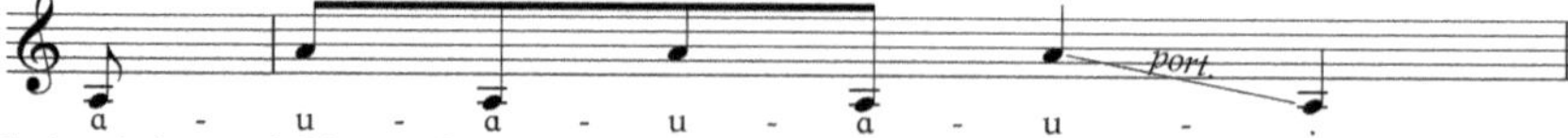

Begin at the lower end of the singer's range, encouraging the voice to flip cleanly into flipped voice as soon as possible. For the u, the throat should be open, while the mouth is rounded into a clear, small 'u' shape. Have the singer yawn while touching their larynx to feel the 'lowness' of the laryngeal posture, then describe the comparative posture change when they flip to build kinesthetic recall of both the released posture and the flip. Bring the lightness down to the last note.

Fig. 10.1 Sample exercises for voice modifications

Balancing Sustainable Singing with Gender-Affirming Modification

Though there is little risk to the client with the three approaches outlined above when principles of healthy voice production are observed, care should be taken to direct enthusiasm, anxiety, or uncertainty into useful action rather than into "pushing" the voice. *Pressed* phonation (particularly where the constrictor muscles are recruited) may provide the singer with temporary aural gains but negative long-term consequences that can evolve into disruptive tension. Other areas that require consideration include:

Onset

Clients may bring phonatory habits from both extremes of this spectrum: hard glottal attacks resulting from attempts to force a brighter sound and overly aspirated onsets. Therapeutic techniques such as straw phonation, *vocal function exercises* (VFE), and *resonant voice* (RV) are useful tools for exploring various onsets. Exercises that work through the vowel sequence with a top-down approach and then descend in pitch are particularly helpful here.

Vocal Fatigue

Clients beginning vocal transition or training after voice injury may struggle with vocal fatigue, particularly when working on troublesome areas of the voice. For these singers, small amounts of practice throughout the day will be far more efficient than longer attempts. Focus should be on reducing any excessive subglottal pressure and tension of the extrinsic musculature. RV, VFE, and *manual circumlaryngeal therapy* (MCT) techniques are critical.

Warm-Up/Cool-Down

The habit of warming up and cooling down the voice at the beginning and ending of the day is a healthy habit for all voice users, but clients struggling with vocal fatigue will find it particularly valuable. SOVT in descending patterns, sirens, or loops works well, including traditional lip trills and fricatives such as [z] or [v].

Laryngeal Positioning

Raised laryngeal position, whether from excessive subglottal pressure, from tension of the extrinsic musculature, or from lip spreading, is often seen in clients wishing to feminize the voice. While a certain amount of lift is acceptable and part of the process, the laryngeal mechanism should never feel "locked," nor should the singer experience soreness when the larynx is palpated. MCT is particularly useful, along with singing exercises where tongue movement and tension are addressed. If SOVTs are used and the laryngeal position relaxes, that may indicate excessive subglottal pressurization; straw phonation or fricatives should be used to improve valving.

Tension and Functional Disruption

Given the incidence of anxiety and mood regulation issues reported in TGNC populations, the likelihood of singers experiencing some level of embodied tension[4] because of these stresses is high. As the voice is a primary communicator of emotional content, it is not surprising that anxiety and concern may translate to vocal tension. Left unchecked, that tension can become disruptive, and therapeutic interventions may be required. The best practice suggests organically including exercises that disrupt tension patterns (tongue out, tongue curled around a pencil or straw, etc.) into the regular warm-up while encouraging clients to report sensations of tightness that might arise[20, 26, 37–41].

Challenges and Other Considerations

Estrogen-Based HRT and The Singing Voice

Although HRT for transfeminine singers does not significantly impact the larger vocal structure, it should not be assumed that there are no effects to consider. Outside of puberty, sex hormones continue to play a role in muscle condition and function, suggesting the possibility that singers undergoing HRT may experience observable shifts in vocal function. There is a lack of research concerning the effects of estrogen on the transitioning singing voice, but existing literature around voice and sports medicine suggests that (a) estrogen may maintain the vocal folds into later life, preventing loss or shift of vocal range that might occur due to the aging process; (b) changes in estrogen and testosterone affect connective tissue and muscle pliability; (c) shifts in estrogen may stimulate or reduce mucosal secretions; and (d) increased estrogen may also influence potential for muscular injury [42–46].

Until further research emerges, it is prudent to make adjustments that take these potential changes into account and encourage the client's physical awareness of their voice, particularly during the first year of HRT. Changes in mucosal secretions may affect hydration or contribute to edema of the vocal folds, requiring monitoring for changes in flexibility, ease of registration, or navigation of *passaggio* points. Increased pliability of the tissue and/or muscle may aid in thinning out the vocal

---

[4] *See* Francis [36].

folds and sustaining a higher tessitura, while increased risk of muscle injury may require airflow and pressure modifications to prevent phonotrauma. The author's clinical observation suggests that fatigue, particularly in the first months of HRT, is also a potential risk. Context is also relevant: Considerations that may be negligible in the avocational singing population can be quite significant to professional voice users.

Anxiety and Mental Health Management

Anxiety around voice, vocal identity, and singing is a significant barrier to progress for singers of any background, but there are unique considerations for the transgender population. Studies report that transgender populations are at higher risk of anxiety-related symptoms and mood disorders, particularly in social contexts; at the same time, musicians (in general) and singers (in particular) are frequently faced with voice and chronic singing-related anxiety [22, 47–49]. Voice-gender incongruence is a significant source of discomfort for transgender and gender-nonconforming individuals in the general population, and that discomfort, a form of social anxiety, is magnified in the singing population [21, 50].

Singing is an intimate, vulnerable activity, and judgment of the voice can feel genuinely dangerous and terrifying. Even if the threat isn't physical, there is still a sense of *perceived* danger, creating a situation where "singers face a degree of risk every time they open their mouths to vocalize" ([22], p. 60). That fear is certainly intensified when judgment of one's singing reflects on the singer's gender identity. There are two facets to this issue: internal friction around voice and self-concept and external conflict around voice and social perception of gender. Singers experience these challenges along a spectrum of intensity which, past a certain point, requires guidance from mental health professionals. Currently, referral to mental healthcare providers for performance anxiety-directed *cognitive-behavioral therapy* (CBT) and/or *desensitization* or *exposure* therapeutic treatment modalities is considered the best practice [49, 51, 52].

Given the barriers to mental health care many singers face, recent studies have investigated potential tools for judicious use by the singing voice professional in the voice studio. *Acceptance and Commitment Coaching* (ACC), based on the associated therapeutic modality, *Acceptance and Commitment Therapy* (ACT), is a promising new area of research. ACT and ACC are not specifically directed at musical or singing-related performance anxiety, but instead address the concept of correcting *psychological inflexibility*: rigid thinking patterns that lead to behavioral processes that may intensify anxious feelings and behavior or prevent the singer from taking actions to either prevent or soothe their own emotional discomfort. While more study is needed, particularly around the complexity of transgender identity and music performance, initial investigations found that teachers who were trained in the ACC modality were able to guide students toward a more flexible approach in their thinking, resulting in improved sense of confidence and agency in their singing and training [51–53].

While the *external* issue of social perception, voice, and gender is a difficult situation, and one beyond the control of any single person, there is much the voice professional can do to help singers resolve the experience of *internal* friction. Current research offers insight into interventions which, used judiciously, may help reduce the anxiety this friction causes. Approaches may include:

(a) Reframing critique as work toward improved *function*, rather than obstacles or criticism of their innate timbre or current sound production.
(b) Incrementally guiding the singer toward a more objective view of their voice, by modeling neutral observations and objective descriptive language when discussing voice.
(c) Identifying and challenging *negative self-talk*, particularly around the voice and its function, and encouraging clients to allow themselves room for stumbles or failure without self-recrimination.
(d) Reducing the emotional cost of errors in performance by focusing on:
    (i) *Risk and threat management*—Simulating stressful experience and practicing responses.
    (ii) *Error management* and *prevention*—Modeling and practicing stress-free attitudes toward errors while minimizing negative consequences of errors through on-the-spot correction.
(e) Kindly but persistently bringing focus back toward the positive qualities of the client's instrument—its expressivity and ability to communicate as well as its natural strengths [18, 22, 51].

Finally, the relationship between voice professional and singer is often emotionally intimate, and, given the frequent lack of access to appropriate mental health care that singers and TGNC individuals face, the voice professional may themselves be in the position of confidante or counselor. Maintaining a balance of supportive care and professionalism without alienating or causing undue anxiety is a delicate line to walk, and the voice professional should take care on how the topic of mental health counseling is broached. A singer's relationship with their voice teacher can be self-affirming, while unconsidered but well-meaning advice from an expert authority figure can unintentionally wreak emotional havoc.

All referrals to therapists should avoid any implication that the singer "needs" therapy because they are TGNC or that being TGNC is inherently traumatic. In the case of professional singers, it may be helpful to approach the subject from the standpoint that careers in the performing arts are stressful in the best of times and that all singers benefit from the guidance of a counselor. For avocational singers, the idea of counseling to live their most authentic life is more likely to be received openly. This is certainly as true for cis-gender singers as it is for TGNC individuals.

Laryngologist, SLP Recommendations, and Access to Care

Much discussion has occurred concerning when and where to recommend singers to seek voice-related health care, and there should be no hesitation in making recommendations to appropriate outside professionals—particularly where the health of the vocal mechanism is concerned. It should also be noted, however, that historically there have been many barriers to comprehensive health care for transgender and performing artist populations. At the time of publication, gender-confirming medical procedures are still not covered by insurance in many locales, and out-of-pocket costs are prohibitive. Even when medical intervention is clearly indicated, the singer may not have the resources to pursue appropriate care or find themselves having to choose between their transition-related medical support and physiological vocal care.

In all cases, voice professionals should reach out and build relationships with the related medical community, to have confidence that the professionals to which they send clients have cultural competency in working with TGNC populations. Beyond that, if the client is unable or resistant to pursuing medical care, one must consider the potential issues the client is facing when considering how to move forward with training. The voice specialist should, in all such cases, explain that vocal training is *habilitative*, rather than *rehabilitative*. While many vocal issues will indubitably benefit from habilitative work, there are many conditions that can be exacerbated by well-meaning habilitative exercises. There is a delicate line to walk in cases where there may be damage or dysfunction, but the singer is unable or unwilling to pursue medical care. In such cases, careful consideration must be given concerning how one should proceed with the client. Transparency around hesitancy can go a long way toward maintaining the client's trust and may reduce reluctance toward outside help. No hard advice can be given, as every individual and situation are different; nevertheless, it is important to remember that a client's perceived reluctance to seek care may stem from significant barriers to access rather than resistance or denial of potential issues.

Conclusion

In the focus on methods and technique, it can be easy to lose sight of the most important aspect of all: transition is a journey, and very few people end up exactly at the destination a person imagines for oneself at the onset of that journey. The voice professional's role is to provide the tools to help clients choose the healthiest routes to travel rather than dictate a precise location. Media narratives of TGNC journeys are often misleading, portraying transition as an inevitable outcome—one in which the person "always knew" and their medical transition was an ordained conclusion, from which they emerged to live happily ever after. Few transitions are that neatly packaged and even the ones which appear seamless from the outside contain doubts, worries, and fears. There may be detours, stops, starts, and more detours. Unsurprisingly, this process is rarely without some level of stress, concern, or even self-doubt.

Singing provides a unique outlet for self-expression, self-soothing, communicating with others, and processing emotional experiences or events for ourselves. For people undergoing the journey of transition, with its myriad stresses and challenges, singing would be an invaluable tool. Yet, many people are shy of using these tools, often due to erroneous beliefs: whether they are "good enough," whether their voice is appropriate for singing, and whether their voice represents who they understand themselves to be. Voice professionals are positioned to help clients unravel those beliefs and gain access to invaluable, authentic self-expression through singing. While building comfort with cultural competency required to work with TGNC singers may seem overwhelming, keeping the ultimate goal in sight—the singers' personal and vocal growth—the work is more than worth the effort.

Appendix 1

Initial Vocal Intake Protocol

What are the vocal outcomes the singer desires? Outcomes should be philosophically specific but functionally open to definition, as desired outcomes may shift as the singer understands their instrument more fully.

What is the singer's current level of experience and vocal ability? This requires both conversation and the performance of singing tasks to fully assess. Listening to the singer speaks will give some indication of their vocal function.

What, if any, impediments to healthy phonation can be identified? Are there functional issues that would need to be addressed regardless of the singer's gender and vocal identity? Potential issues such as tension patterns, posture imbalance, breath pressure, resonance, and articulation may be quietly noted before any singing tasks are undertaken simply by observing and listening to the singer's spoken phonation.

What are the direct and indirect causes of such impediments? This is where knowledge of their background will be useful. Habits and activities that may lead to physiological damage or phonotrauma, such as smoking, work, or recreation in loud environments or even jobs that are vocally demanding, should be noted.

What interventions and training goals will address both the singer's personal goals and any observed vocal impediments? A TGNC singer, regardless of their gender-related vocal goals, is still a *singer*—a voice user to whom a voice professional's first responsibility is the development and maintenance of healthy phonatory habits.

Which tools will be used to address the determined training goals? Clients deserve transparency concerning the directions in which the voice specialist intends to explore with their voice. Even if the client has little to no knowledge of vocal function, simple but clear explanations of the "whys and wherefores" of what they are being asked to do significantly increase compliance.

References

1. Jahn A, Blitzer A. A short history of laryngoscopy. Logoped Phoniatr Vocol. 1996;21:181–5. https://earandvoicedoctor.com/media/Short_History_of_Laryngoscopy.pdf
2. Miller R. Historical overview of voice pedagogy. In: Sataloff RT, editor. Vocal health and pedagogy: science, assessment, and treatment. San Diego, CA: Plural; 2017a. p. 11–23.
3. Miller R. The singing teacher in the age of voice science. In: Sataloff RT, editor. Vocal health and pedagogy: science, assessment, and treatment. San Diego, CA: Plural; 2017b. p. 7–10.
4. Graham FA. He said, she said, they said: making the case for a gender neutral pedagogy. VoicePrints. 2018;15(5):87–91.
5. Cayari C, Graham FA, Jampole EJ, O'Leary J. Trans voices speak: suggestions from trans educators about working with trans students. Music Educat J. 2021;108(1):50–6.
6. Clarkson NL. Teaching trans students, teaching trans studies. Fem Teach. 2017;27(2-3):233–52. https://doi.org/10.5406/femteacher.27.2-3.0233.
7. Phillips KH, Williams J, Edwin R. The young singer. In: McPherson GE, Welch GF, editors. The oxford handbook of music education, vol. 1. Oxford: Oxford University Press; 2012. https://doi.org/10.1093/oxfordhb/9780199730810.013.0036_update_001.
8. Kozan AL, Hammond SC. The singing voice. In: Adler RK, Hirsch S, Pickering J, editors. Voice and communication therapy for the transgender/gender diverse client: a comprehensive clinical guide. San Diego, CA: Plural Publishing, Inc; 2018. p. 291–334.
9. Bos N. Teaching transgender and gender non-conforming singers. VoicePrints. 2017;14(3):6–7. https://search.proquest.com/openview/6300f2009ffe25db29a77c9feb214565/1?pq-origsite=gscholar&cbl=2069483
10. Davies S. Training the transgender singer: finding the voice inside. Inter Nos(Spring) 2016: 10–11. https://www.nats.org/_Library/Independent_Voices_Articles/training_transgender_singer-10-2016.pdf
11. Jackson Hearns, L., & Kremer, B. (2018). The singing teacher's guide to transgender voices. Plural Publishing Incorporated San Diego, CA. https://ebookcentral.proquest.com/lib/gbv/detail.action?docID=5676540.
12. Lessley E. Teaching transgender singers [Dissertation]. University of Washington. 2017. https://digital.lib.washington.edu/researchworks/bitstream/handle/1773/40272/Lessley_washington_0250E_17535.pdf?sequence=1
13. Sauerland W. Legitimate voices: a multi-case study of trans and non-binary singers in the applied voice studio [Dissertation]. Teachers College. 2018. https://academiccommons.columbia.edu/doi/10.7916/D87D4BPZ/download.
14. Heinz M. Communicating while transgender: apprehension, loneliness, and willingness to communicate in a Canadian sample. SAGE Open. 2018;8(2):215824401877778. https://doi.org/10.1177/2158244018777780.
15. Blackwell J, Miksza P, Evans P, McPherson GE. Student vitality, teacher engagement, and rapport in studio music instruction. Front Psychol. 2020;11:1007. https://doi.org/10.3389/fpsyg.2020.01007.

16. Clemmons J. The importance of being earnest: rapport in the applied studio—college music symposium. College Music Symposium, 49 2009. . https://symposium.music.org/index.php/49/item/9224-the-importance-of-being-earnest-rapport-in-the-applied-studio
17. Mackworth-Young L. Pupil-centred learning in piano lessons: an evaluated action-research programme focusing on the psychology of the individual. Psychol Music. 1990;18(1):73–86. https://doi.org/10.1177/0305735690181006.
18. Graham FA. Singing while female: a narrative study on gender, identity & experience of female voice in cis, transmasculine & non-binary singers. Ed.D.C.T. Teachers College, Columbia University. 2019. https://doi.org/10.7916/d8-mnh1-st58.
19. Sataloff RT, editor. Vocal health and pedagogy: science, assessment, and treatment. 3rd ed. San Diego, CA: Plural; 2017.
20. Titze IR, Verdolini Abbott K. Vocology: the science and practice of voice habilitation. Salt Lake City: National Center for Voice and Speech; 2012.
21. Abril CR. I have a voice but I just can't sing: a narrative investigation of singing and social anxiety. Music Educ Res. 2007;9(1):1–15. https://doi.org/10.1080/14613800601127494.
22. Barefield R. Fear of singing: identifying and assisting singers with chronic anxiety issues. Music Educ J. 2012;98(3):60–3. http://www.jstor.org/stable/41433281
23. Casals A, Vilar M, Ayats J. 'I'm not sure if I can. . But I want to sing!' research on singing as a soloist through the art of improvising verses. Br J Music Educ. 2011;28(3):247–61. https://doi.org/10.1017/S0265051711000192.
24. Hendricks KS. The sources of self-efficacy. Update: applications of research in music. Education. 2016;35(1):32–8. https://doi.org/10.1177/8755123315576535.
25. Hogle LA. Fostering singing agency through emotional differentiation in an inclusive singing environment. Res Stud Music Educ. 2020;43(2):179–94. https://doi.org/10.1177/1321103X20930426.
26. Titze IR, Palaparthi A, Cox K, Stark A, Maxfield L, Manternach B. Vocalization with semi-occluded airways is favorable for optimizing sound production. PLoS Comput Biol. 2021;17(3):e1008744. https://doi.org/10.1371/journal.pcbi.1008744.
27. Abrahams F. The application of critical pedagogy to music teaching and learning. Visions of research in music education. 2005. 6. http://users.rider.edu/~vrme/v6n1/visions/Abrahams%20The%20Application%20of%20Critical%20Pedagogy.pdf
28. Taetle L, Cutietta R. Learning theories as roots of current musical practice and research. In: Colwell R, Richardson C, editors. The new handbook of research on music teaching and learning: a project of the music educators national conference. Oxford: Oxford University Press; 2012.
29. Chapman JL. Singing and teaching singing: a holistic approach to classical voice. 3rd ed. San Diego, CA: Plural Publishing; 2017.
30. Czajkowski A-ML, Greasley AE, Allis M. Mindfulness for musicians: a mixed methods study investigating the effects of 8-week mindfulness courses on music students at a leading conservatoire. Music Sci. 2020;26(2):259–79. https://doi.org/10.1177/1029864920941570.
31. Parncutt R, McPherson G, editors. The science & psychology of music performance: creative strategies for teaching and learning. Oxford: Oxford University Press; 2002. http://site.ebrary.com/lib/academiccompletetitles/home.action
32. Carew L, Dacakis G, Oates J. The effectiveness of oral resonance therapy on the perception of femininity of voice in male-to-female transsexuals. J Voice. 2007;21(5):591–603. https://doi.org/10.1016/j.jvoice.2006.05.005.
33. Dahl KL, Mahler LA. Acoustic features of transfeminine voices and perceptions of voice femininity. J Voice. 2020;34(6):961.e19–26. https://doi.org/10.1016/j.jvoice.2019.05.012.
34. Titze IR. Physiologic and acoustic differences between male and female voices. J Acoust Soc Am. 1989;85(4):1699–707. https://doi.org/10.1121/1.397959.
35. Wiltshire A. Not by pitch alone: a view of transsexual vocal rehabilitation. Natl Stud Speech Lang Hearing Assoc J. 1995;22:53–7. https://pubs.asha.org/doi/pdf/10.1044/nsshla_22_53

36. Francis AL. The embodied theory of stress: a constructionist perspective on the experience of stress. Rev Gen Psychol. 2018;22(4):398–405. https://doi.org/10.1037/gpr0000164.
37. Bane M, Brown M, Angadi V, Croake DJ, Andreatta RD, Stemple JC. Vocal function exercises for normal voice: with and without semi-occlusion. Int J Speech Lang Pathol. 2019;21(2):175–81. https://doi.org/10.1080/17549507.2017.1416176.
38. Guzman M. Semioccluded vocal tract exercises: a physiologic approach for voice training and therapy [Dissertation]. University of Tampere, Tampere, Finland. 2017. https://trepo.tuni.fi/bitstream/handle/10024/100627/978-952-03-0391-4.pdf?sequence=7&isAllowed=y.
39. Guzman M, Laukkanen A-M, Krupa P, Horáček J, Švec JG, Geneid A. Vocal tract and glottal function during and after vocal exercising with resonance tube and straw. J Voice. 2013;27(4):523.e19–34. https://doi.org/10.1016/j.jvoice.2013.02.007.
40. Jafari N, Salehi A, Izadi F, Talebian Moghadam S, Ebadi A, Dabirmoghadam P, Faham M, Shahbazi M. Vocal function exercises for muscle tension dysphonia: auditory-perceptual evaluation and self-assessment rating. J Voice. 2017;31(4):506.e25–31. https://doi.org/10.1016/j.jvoice.2016.10.009.
41. Sandage MJ, Hoch M. Exercise physiology: Perspective for vocal training. pp. 847–851.
42. Chidi-Ogbolu N, Baar K. Effect of estrogen on musculoskeletal performance and injury risk. Front Physiol. 2018;9:1834. https://doi.org/10.3389/fphys.2018.01834.
43. Gugatschka M, Kiesler K, Obermayer-Pietsch B, Schoekler B, Schmid C, Groselj-Strele A, Friedrich G. Sex hormones and the elderly male voice. J Voice. 2010;24(3):369–73. https://doi.org/10.1016/j.jvoice.2008.07.004.
44. Kumar H, Garg A, Ajai Chandra NS, Singh SP, Datta R. Voice and endocrinology. Indian J Endocrinol Metab. 2016;20(5):590–4. https://doi.org/10.4103/2230-8210.190523.
45. Ouyoung LM, Villegas BC, Liu C, Talmor G, Sinha UK. Effects of resonance voice therapy on hormone-related vocal disorders in professional singers: a pilot study. Clin Med Insights Ear Nose Throat. 2018;11:1–7. https://doi.org/10.1177/1179550618786934.
46. Rodney JP, Sataloff RT. The effects of hormonal contraception on the voice: history of its evolution in the literature. J Voice. 2016;30(6):726–30. https://doi.org/10.1016/j.jvoice.2015.08.014.
47. Bouman WP, Claes L, Brewin N, Crawford JR, Millet N, Fernandez-Aranda F, Arcelus J. Transgender and anxiety: a comparative study between transgender people and the general population. Int J Transg. 2017;18(1):16–26. https://doi.org/10.1080/15532739.2016.1258352.
48. Millet N, Longworth J, Arcelus J. Prevalence of anxiety symptoms and disorders in the transgender population: a systematic review of the literature. Int J Transg. 2017;18(1):27–38. https://doi.org/10.1080/15532739.2016.1258353.
49. Wilson GD, Roland D. Performance anxiety. In: Parncutt R, McPherson G, editors. The science & psychology of music performance: creative strategies for teaching and learning. Oxford: Oxford University Press; 2002. p. 47–62. https://doi.org/10.1093/acprof:oso/9780195138108.001.0001.
50. Kennedy E, Thibeault SL. Voice-gender incongruence and voice health information-seeking behaviors in the transgender community. Am J Speech Lang Pathol. 2020;29(3):1563–73. https://doi.org/10.1044/2020_AJSLP-19-00188.
51. Kenny D. The psychology of music performance anxiety. Oxford: OUP Oxford; 2011.
52. Shaw TA, Juncos DG, Winter D. Piloting a new model for treating music performance anxiety: training a singing teacher to use acceptance and commitment coaching with a student. Front Psychol. 2020;11:882. https://doi.org/10.3389/fpsyg.2020.00882.
53. Juncos DG, Heinrichs GA, Towle P, Duffy K, Grand SM, Morgan MC, Smith JD, Kalkus E. Acceptance and commitment therapy for the treatment of music performance anxiety: a pilot study with student vocalists. Front Psychol. 2017;8:986. https://doi.org/10.3389/fpsyg.2017.00986.

Chapter 11
Behavioral Management for Masculinization of Voice and Communication Across the Gender Spectrum

Olivia Boddicker and Rachel Kominsky

Introduction

Transgender and gender non-conforming (TGNC) individuals often identify voice as a key factor contributing to their gender dysphoria and as an identifier that causes others to misgender them both in person and over the telephone. Within the TGNC population, transmasculine can be used as an umbrella term for individuals assigned female at birth (AFAB) who have a masculine and/or non-binary identity [1]. These clients are quoted as approximately 25% of the TGNC population [2]. This group has often been overlooked as one that would benefit from voice therapy, as exogenous androgen therapy has been found to lower fundamental frequency or pitch. However, results of androgen therapy are variable and still incompletely understood. Additionally, understanding the complexity of voice as it relates to gender makes it clear that beyond pitch there are gendered patterns of speech, voice, and communication that could be targeted in therapy and facilitate a more gender congruent outcome for the client. Research has shown that when a TGNC individual's voice is congruent with their gender expression, they report greater well-being, specifically higher quality of life, self-esteem, and lower levels of anxiety and depression [3]. For these reasons, voice therapy for the transmasculine client has been the subject of research, development, and practice in recent years. This chapter will review androgen therapy's effect on voice, discuss characteristics of voice often

O. Boddicker
Department of Otolaryngology, Grabscheid Voice and Swallowing Center of Mount Sinai, New York, NY, USA
e-mail: olivia.boddicker@mountsinai.org

R. Kominsky (✉)
Division of Laryngology, Department of Otorhinolaryngology—Head and Neck Surgery, Montefiore Medical Center, Bronx, NY, USA
e-mail: rkominsky@montefiore.org

M. S. Courey et al. (eds.), *Voice and Communication in Transgender and Gender Diverse Individuals*, https://doi.org/10.1007/978-3-031-24632-6_11

associated with the masculine side of the gender spectrum, review specific therapy techniques that facilitate congruence with a masculine identity, and describe challenges that may arise when working with the transmasculine or TGNC client wishing to masculinize their voice.

Effects of Testosterone on the Voice

The effects of external androgen therapy, testosterone, on the voice have been studied for decades, with more research occurring over the past 20 years. It is thought that the same physiological changes that occur in the larynx during puberty occur when an individual takes testosterone, namely, that the vocal folds increase in mass, and the changes are irreversible [4]. Multiple retrospective studies, admittedly with small sample sizes, have shown a decrease in fundamental frequency with testosterone therapy [2].

There have been few prospective studies regarding timing and degree of voice deepening after starting testosterone. Some retrospective studies suggest voice changes begin within 2–4 months [2, 5]. However, more recent prospective studies have shown that the first significant changes in speaking fundamental frequency can occur within 2 weeks of initiating testosterone therapy, and within 9 months, these clients can reach a fundamental frequency equal to cisgender males [6]. In a study by Nygren which followed transmasculine clients taking testosterone for 24 months, the largest drop in pitch was seen in the first 2–5 months with no significant decrease from 12 to 24 months [7]. Cosyns et al. showed that 38 transmasculine clients who were on androgen therapy for at least 2 years were, as a group, indistinguishable from cisgender male controls in pitch, intonation, and perturbation. Interestingly, it was concluded that approximately 10% of transmasculine individuals will have pitch-lowering difficulties, which is thought to be associated with diminished androgen sensitivity [8]. Given that not all individuals' fundamental frequency is affected in the same way or to the same extent by testosterone, this leaves a role for clients to work with voice specialists to achieve their desired goals. Voice clinicians should consider the wide range of goals within the transmasculine TGNC group and the need to this diversity when it comes to the desired voice [1].

Despite the focus on low fundamental frequency as an indicator of vocal maleness, Van Borsel et al. performed a study in 2009 to rate maleness of speakers and found no correlation between fundamental frequency and listener perception of maleness [9]. It was hypothesized that an absence of correlation between average fundamental frequency and rating of maleness could mean that in TGNC individuals wishing to have a masculine-sounding voice, fundamental frequency is a less important factor for gender expression compared to transfeminine and TGNC individuals wishing to have a feminine sounding voice. It could also reflect a more general societal trend that a male with a higher pitch voice is more accepted than a lower-pitch voice in females.

There have been attempts to determine how testosterone affects voice measures beyond pitch in transmasculine individuals. Hancock et al. [10] studied seven transgender males prospectively during initiation of testosterone therapy over a 1-year period. Voice and self-perception measures were recorded at 3-month intervals up to 1 year. While the transgender men did have lower pitch, they showed wide variation in phonation frequency range, 57% of participants with increased and 43% with decreased range. However, the change was only statistically significant in one participant (who increased in range). It was also noted that it was insufficient to collect acoustic measures alone without including self-perception measures of voice, as the objective measures did not always correspond with voice satisfaction.

Vocal Dissatisfaction in Individuals Post-Testosterone

Many transmasculine and TGNC individuals are pleased with their voice after testosterone therapy, though there is a growing body of research that indicates it is not always sufficient to produce correct perception of one's gender and may lead to difficulties in vocal function. Van Borsel et al. [2] found that in a study of 16 transgender male individuals who had taken testosterone for 1 year, 25% were inconsistently "addressed as a woman" by strangers due at least in part to their voice. This is not a completely unexpected result. In their 2009 study examining the importance of pitch and resonance in gender perception, Hillenbrand and Clark found that changing only pitch or resonance alone is not sufficient to reliably change listener attribution of a speaker's gender. Furthermore, being misgendered is not the only aspect of voice that may concern a TGNC individual. In their 2021 study, Azul, Hancock, and Nygren [11] conducted interviews with 14 German-speaking, gender-diverse AFAB individuals; 54% of participants stated that testosterone had restricted at least one aspect of vocal function, with the most common being voice quality, vocal control/stability, pitch range, vocal endurance, and vocal power/projection. Considering that these restrictions echo the findings of existing studies [12; Nygren et al. 7], further research is warranted in regard to the satisfaction and function of transmasculine and TGNC voice after exposure to testosterone. The transmasculine and TGNC client's entire "vocal situation" must be taken into account when treated by healthcare professionals, not simply lowering of fundamental frequency.

The term "vocal situation," utilized by Azul in 2015 [1], encompasses all factors, internal and external, that affect the voice. This includes but is not limited to the three domains discussed in Azul et al. [12] and Chennupati [13]: voice function (the capacity to meet vocal demands), sociocultural positioning (the understanding and portrayal of one's position/role in social and cultural contexts), and communication-related well-being (balance of psychological, social, and emotional stressors versus resources). This framework provides a holistic approach through which voice and communication specialists (speech-language pathologists, laryngologists, voice coaches, voice trainers, singing teachers, and more) can identify and therefore better serve the needs of transmasculine and TGNC individuals.

Masculine Voice and Communication

To guide clients seeking voice masculinization with or without having been exposed to testosterone, first a definition of "masculine voice" and a "masculine communication style" must be established. Cisgender male voices and communication are often described as having a lower pitch, "chest resonance," increased vocal intensity (loudness), decreased pitch variation, downward-sloping intonation patterns, less-precise articulation, and a more stoic facial expression. However, these are often simplifications of a more complex understanding of the male voice and communication style.

Pitch

Fundamental frequency (F0) is often regarded by specialists and laypeople alike as one of the most salient characteristics of communication that informs the gender of the speaker [14–16]. In their 2009 study, Hillenbrand and Clark utilized a source-filter synthesizer to shift the fundamental frequency and/or formants of 25 sentences each recorded by cisgender men and women and played for 21 typical-hearing speech-language pathology students. They found that shifting F0 into cisgender female and male ranges resulted in 34.3% of cismale samples identified as female and 19.1% of cisfemale samples identified as male.

While the above studies have shown that changing the fundamental frequency of speech can result in a change in speaker gender identification, speaking with pitch in the traditionally male range does not guarantee that a speaker will be identified as male. Gelfer and Bennett's study in [17] showed that even when the speaker's F0 when reading passages and phrases was shifted into typical cismale and cisfemale ranges, 49.3% of cismale voices were identified as male with the highest F0 at 207 Hz and 85.0% of cisfemale voices continued to be identified as female with the lowest F0 at 116 Hz. Wolfe et al. demonstrated that within a cohort of 20 transfeminine individuals, the lowest F0 of an individual who identified as female was 155 Hz, well below the typical cisfemale range, and the highest F0 of a speaker who identified as male was 145 Hz.

Additionally, vocal pitch does not exist in a vacuum; language and culture have a demonstrable effect on F0 of the speaker. In a literature review of cismale pitch across languages, it was reported that between British English and Urdu, there is shown a 10.7 semitone, (a linear measure of mean F0 based on half steps in musical notation, used for comparison across the frequency range) difference in F0 [18]. Even within American English, in a study ($N = 200$) examining the F0 of Black individuals within spontaneous speech and a reading task, a 2 semitone (ST) difference in women and 1 ST difference in men were noted when compared with F0 norms for white individuals in the United States of America [19].

The term "male pitch" encompasses a wide range of semitones, particularly when examined globally. This variation in F0 norm, as shown above, results in unreliable identification of a speaker's sex and/or gender. However, when F0 is modified in conjunction with formant frequency, a marked increase in changing perception of gender is observed [17, 20–23].

Resonance and Articulation

Resonance can be thought of as the quality, tone, or color of the voice that comes from source-filter interaction when the vibrations produced by the vocal folds travel along the vocal tract. Adjectives often associated with masculine-sounding voices are "full," "bass-y," "deep," "resonant," and "chest focused," among others. Vocal quality is informed by the spacing of harmonics and formants above the speaker's F0. In voices rated as male, the first three vowel formants are found to be more closely spaced together and lower in pitch than those of voices rated as female [21, 24, 25]. Specifically, both Munson [26] and Avery and Liss [27] found that perceived voice masculinity was inversely related to the frequency of the second formant in cismales. Though there was significant overlap in the ranges of vowel formant frequencies for /ɑ/ and /i/ in cisfemale and cismale subjects, a 2013 study by Gelfer and Bennett ($N = 30$) demonstrated there was a statistically significant difference between cismen and ciswomen. Additionally, in a study examining perception of masculinity or femininity at the word level ($N = 44$), participants were more often rated as masculine when saying words that have "back vowels" such as /u/, /o/, and /oʊ/, suggesting a correlation between posterior-focused resonance and increased perception of masculinity [26]. No perceptual correlates (e.g., "deep," "chest voice," "resonant," etc.) were assigned to any of the above findings by their authors or participants.

Formants are dictated by the shape of the vocal tract, and there is data to support that differences in articulation can affect the perception of a speaker's gender. In addition to differences in the formation of /i/ and /ɑ/, there are differences noted in the spectral signal of /s/ and to a lesser-studied extent, /ʃ/. In a 1996 study examining the degree of masculinity in subjects' voices ($N = 35$), those that were classified as less masculine sounding to female listeners demonstrated a higher-frequency center for /s/ and a less diffuse energy distribution when producing /ʃ/ [27]. These differences are produced with more lip spreading and lip rounding, respectively. There is limited evidence to suggest that cismales with "clearer" speech and articulatory precision are perceived with a greater degree of femininity [28]. However, further research is required to support the role of articulation in gender perception [14, 29].

Similar to fundamental frequency, resonance patterns, and articulation, vowel formant frequencies are different across speakers who speak the same language, but do not come from similar linguistic and/or cultural backgrounds. For example, in vowels common across both languages (/i/, /ɛ/, and /ɪ/), native German speakers were found to produce the vowels with significantly different spectral signals as compared to native English speakers [30]. Similarly, when examining the production of /u/ in native English and French speakers, Flege [31] found there was a higher and more variable second formant frequency in native English speakers. These differences should be considered when working with clients of multiple linguistic and varied cultural backgrounds.

In summation, research demonstrates that masculine-identified speech tends to have lower pitch and lower and less-spaced formant frequencies, affecting perception of vocal resonance and articulation. Even so, Assmann et al. [20] found that when resonance and pitch are shifted, listeners were still more likely to identify cismale voice samples as male and cisfemale samples as female, citing "residual indicators of voice gender" as a possible explanation.

Intonation, Pitch Variation, and Volume

Other cited perceptual correlates of vocal masculinity include a downward-sloping intonation pattern, and a "monotone" speaking pattern, or reduced pitch variability.

In their 1990 study, Wolfe et al. examined the spontaneous speech samples of 40 individuals (20 transfeminine individuals and 20 cisgender male and female college students). The samples were played for speech-language pathology students, who were then asked to rate them as male or female, as well as the degree of masculinity and femininity in speech. Male-rated speakers demonstrated less use of upward intonation, more extensive downward intonation, and more frequent instances of level shifts (shift between terminal pitch of previous utterance and initial pitch of subsequent utterance of less than 5 Hz) and level intonation. The mean extent of upward intonation for both male- and female-rated speakers was 2.5 ST; that is to say, while the frequency of upward intonation usage was less for male-rated speakers, the pitch change was similar in comparison with female-rated speakers. In contrast is Avery and Liss' study [27], in which they found more masculine speech had the same number of "ups" as less masculine speech and a lesser range of semitones utilized. Hancock et al. also found in 2014 that masculine-rated voices utilized a slightly smaller range in pitch than feminine-rated voice, but the difference between the two was insignificant. These conflicting results reflect the variability and complexity of speech patterns. The evidence supports that extensive downward shifts in pitch are identified as a masculine speaking pattern; however, the stereotype of a monotone, unchanging male voice, is not.

Similarly, there are limited data to suggest that males exhibit a greater average vocal intensity than females [32]. There is a weak correlation between femininity and decreased vocal intensity [33], as well as with the descriptors "light" and "soft." However, it has been shown that these adjectives do not correlate with decreased sound pressure level (SPL). Further study is needed to determine the role of vocal intensity and masculinity.

Language and Nonverbal Communication

As communication specialists providing gender-affirming care, it is important to address the entirety of a person's communication style as it aligns with their communication goals. This would include diction, pragmatics, and body language that is incongruent with the client's gender. The stereotype that men are assertive or commanding is a feature that can be communicated in verbal and nonverbal language. Assertiveness is a trait that is traditionally associated with people in positions of power. Largely, throughout the course of history, that role has been assigned to men [34]. In a meta-analysis, Leaper and Ayres [35] examined assertive language, thought to be more masculine, in opposition with affiliative language, which is thought to be more feminine. They define affiliative language as functioning to affirm or positively engage one's conversational partner (e.g., showing support, expressing agreement, acknowledging the other's contributions), whereas assertive language functions to advance one's personal agency (e.g., directive statements, giving information, disagreeing with or criticizing the other's contributions). They found that men tended to and were more likely to use assertive language than women and that women tended to use more affiliative language.

Carli [36] found that people who used tentative language, regardless of their gender, were rated as less powerful, competent, and intelligent than their direct language counterparts.

In their 2009 study, Palomares sought to link these findings to specific genders and examined the use of tentative language by women and men. Tentative language was defined by the use of hedges ("sort of," "might," "kinda," "probably"), disclaimers ("I'm not sure," "I don't know," "you should double check," "I may be wrong"), and questions tagged onto statements ("right?," "do you agree?," "isn't it?"). University students ($N = 276$) identifying as either men or women were asked to write an email to a random recipient, responding to a question about a given topic. They were given only a name (John or Jennifer) of their recipient and told they would receive responses later in the quarter. Palomares randomly assigned topics that were stereotypically masculine, feminine, and gender neutral to each participant. He found that the amount of tentative language used was not a function of a specific gender, but rather was dependent on the group dynamics. Women were more likely to use tentative language when writing about a "masculine" topic to recipients named John (intergroup), but when speaking to Jennifer (intragroup), tentativeness was not increased. The same was true of male participants, an increase in tentative language was noted for "feminine" topics in an intergroup context, but not for intragroup contexts. Both female and male participants used the same amount of tentative language when speaking about gender-neutral topics in both group contexts [37].

A similar relationship to power and status, rather than gender, emerges when examining nonverbal communication. There is evidence to support the idea that women display more affiliative nonverbal communication, such as more frequent smiling, increased head tilting, and nods [38, 39] however, this may be mediated by the fact that people who are perceived as less dominant are expected to smile more [40]. In their meta-analysis, Hall, Coats, and LeBeau found that people of higher status take up more physical space and exhibit a more open posture. Most notably, however, they found that nonverbal communication is highly heterogeneous, particularly when examined through the lens of power and status. Additional mediators of nonverbal communication are inter- vs intragroup context, familiarity with communication partners, culture, and country of the speaker [38, 41, 42].

Treatment: Techniques and Strategies for Communication and Voice Masculinization

Upon examination of gender and communication, one clear theme emerges: how one performs and expresses their gender is informed by context. Gender expression is a broad and diverse spectrum and must be treated as such in a therapeutic setting. Operating from the lens of individualized, trauma-informed, and client-centered care means the client, not the clinician, sets their goals for voice and communication. This helps ensure clinicians are meeting the individual needs of each client.

The techniques and strategies for voice masculinization listed in the following section are intended for use with clients of any gender identity wishing to add an element of perceived masculinity to their voice. The client should feel encouraged to choose any or all aspects of communication that allows them to achieve congruency with their gender identity and feel most authentic to themselves. Clinicians should present the possible treatment targets in the initial evaluation, providing examples of each, and develop a plan of care that addresses the client's priorities.

At present, there is a paucity of empirical evidence and research into specific techniques for voice masculinization, and as such practice is disproportionately guided by clinical expertise [43–46]. The following techniques are intended to provide ideas for treatment and should be critically evaluated before use to determine efficacy and relevancy to each individual client.

Pitch

The process of habituating a pitch different from one's native F0 requires careful consideration of vocal health and sustainability. The voice specialist works with the client on achieving a voice that does not cause strain, pain, or fatigue. This applies in cases of elevating or lowering pitch.

The selection of a target F0 is informed by the client's maximum phonational frequency range (the range from lowest to highest pitch an individual can produce) combined with the client's report of vocal comfort. As with vocal feminization for

TGNC individuals, choosing a pitch that is not the client's absolute lowest vocalized pitch allows for naturalistic intonation contours, sustainability, and extensive falling intonation that has been noted to influence perception of masculinity in voice. Gelfer and Mordaunt [47] suggest a conversational speaking range of 12 ST in total. Clinicians may elect to select a pitch that is at least 2.5 semitones below the top of a selected speaking range [48], allowing for sufficient rising and falling intonation. If a sufficiently low pitch is not yet vocally comfortable for the client to produce consistently, muscle tension and vocal flexibility may need to be addressed first. Warming up by performing descending pitch glides that extend beneath the target F0 is recommended, as are ascending glides that extend above the target F0 in voice feminization.

Choosing a target pitch:

1. Utilize frequency tracing software (Visi-Pitch) or apps (Pitch Analyst, Voice Tools) to determine the client's MPFR; for example, 110–420 Hz.
2. Calculate a pitch range that is 12 ST in length within the client's MPFR that is low but comfortable for the client to access consistently. For this example, that might be 120–254 Hz (12 ST).
3. Choose a pitch that is *at least* 2.5 ST below the top of the speaking range. In this case, for a client wanting a lower pitch, it may be more than 2.5 ST below or 140 Hz.
4. If the client is not yet comfortable producing this pitch consistently, choose a higher pitch, and as sessions progress, you can gradually drop the pitch as tolerated.

Pitch can be addressed directly or indirectly depending on the attitudes and feelings of the client. A commonly used method of direct pitch work is targeting F0 by monitoring pitch over time with frequency tracing software, most often in the form of a phone application (app). Some clients may be negatively impacted by focusing on a numerical goal or monitoring themselves on a pitch app. Others may find the use of such apps helpful and facilitative of generalization, as has been shown in research with AMAB transfeminine individuals [49].

The use of an anchor pitch marked by a note name (e.g., D3) as opposed to the acoustic correlate in Hz (D3 = 146.83 Hz) may be beneficial for clients to reduce the effects of stigmatization and self-judgment that can arise when working with pitch in Hz. The pitch is played by the client or clinician and then hummed before moving directly into speech. The hum can be replaced with other SOVT sounds such as /z/, /v/, and /ð/ or voiced trill to best address the needs of the client:

1. Using a pitch app, pitch pipe, or piano, play the chosen anchor pitch.
2. Ask the client to produce the pitch using an SOVT sound, such as /z/, /v/, and /ð/. Alternatively, if the client is working on other aspects of voice (airflow, muscular relaxation, etc.), the clinician may choose another sound on which the client can produce the anchor pitch to target multiple goals at once.

3. After the client begins to repeatedly produce the chosen sound on the anchor pitch, guide them to move fluently from the sound into a speech ("mmmhello" "mmmmy name is Alex"). Clinicians can level-set difficulty of stimuli (word, phrase, sentence, etc.) in accordance with the client's needs.
4. It may be helpful at first to begin with chanted speech (speaking on the anchor pitch, no breaks, variation, or intonation), until adequate airflow, freedom in sound, and an ideal pitch are maintained. Then, more naturalistic intonation and pitch variation can be introduced.

In her 2021 dissertation, François, using a treatment protocol of circumlaryngeal massage and reposturing during phonation, found a significant effect of a lower F0 and a longer vocal tract in transmasculine participants ($N = 15$).

Step 1: Circumlaryngeal Massage

- 1.5 min of sternocleidomastoid pull downs
- 3.5 min of thyrohyoid space anterior-posterior massage
- 2.5 min of circular anterior-posterior massage of the suprahyoid muscle
- 1.5 min of dynamic lateral stretches of the thyroid cartilage
- 2 min of static lateral stretches of the thyroid cartilage (60-s displacement to each side)
- 2 min of laryngeal pull downs
- 2 min of hyoid pull downs
- *Step 2: Laryngeal Reposturing with Voicing*
- SLP administers thyroid pull downs and hyoid pushbacks, examining voice quality after each posture. This can be achieved by having the client briefly speak after each posture and then deciding which movement results in an ideal voice—without strain.
- SLP teaches client to self-administer reposturing technique(s).
- SLP guides client through a hierarchy of speech (see "Resonance" section for description of general hierarchy) with /m/ as facilitator. Over time, the participant is instructed to stop manual depression and attempt to maintain the posture and quality of the voice.
- If client has difficulty maintaining the voice quality, SLP offers verbal cues to maintain new voice, such as "think to yawn slightly, have a somewhat elongated jaw, use /m/ when needed."
- SLP prompts client to give a name to the new voice ("back voice, goal voice, new voice, throat voice") and utilizes negative practice between baseline and target voices with the client's chosen label [50]

As vocal tract length was correlated with a decrease in the third and fourth formants, this protocol may also result in a more masculine resonance pattern as well. If the clinician feels that directly targeting pitch is not ideal for the client, a lower pitch may be indirectly realized as a secondary effect of resonance training as evidenced above.

Resonance

Due to the lack of research supporting specific treatment methods to target resonance, the most valuable tool of the clinician is a well-trained ear and intimate knowledge of anatomy and physiology of the voice. As previously stated, there is evidence supporting relatively low and close spacing of the first three formant frequencies to produce a voice that is more often perceived as masculine. "Formants" are modified by changing the shape of the vocal tract (velum, tongue, jaw opening, etc.). As such, sound quality can be altered by modifying the vocal fold configuration and/or the vocal tract (formants).

As above, Munson [26] found that spoken words with "back vowels" (/u/, /o/, /ɑ/, /ɔ/) were more often rated as masculine. This is possibly due to the longer vocal tract size found in taller individuals, which often includes cismales. Therefore, there may be an indication for utilization of "back vowels" as facilitators of clustering formant frequencies in resonance. As in traditional resonant voice therapy, prompting the client to produce, reflect on, and describe the physical sensation they experience when producing these vowel sounds can be helpful:

1. Establish a baseline by asking the client to describe where they normally feel their voice when speaking.
2. On a comfortable pitch or target pitch, ask the client to produce different "back vowels" (/u/, /o/, /ɑ/, /ɔ/) and describe how it differs or is similar to their baseline voice and the previous sounds ("Was that feeling the *same* or *different* than the /u/ sound from before? How so? Same or different feeling than the voice you walked in with?"). Move between sounds as necessary to allow for sufficient exploration of sensations.
3. Choose which sound is most facilitative of an ideal resonance based on client descriptors, preferences, and clinician's trained ear.
4. Move through hierarchy of generalization (see below), gradually introducing more "front vowels" (/i/, /ɛ/, /e/, /æ/) when client is able to consistently produce the ideal resonance with "back vowels." Pay attention specifically to the color of front vowels to monitor for change in placement. Cue with client's placement descriptors as needed.

In *The Voice Book for Trans and Non-Binary People*, Mills and Stoneham [51] advocate for voice masculinization treatment targets of chest and pharyngeal resonance, which involve a relatively low larynx position, release at the base of tongue, and release in the jaw. Suggested facilitating techniques include (pp. 119–121):

1. "Yawn talk": pretending to yawn and speaking into the space
2. Voice wobbling: clasping the hands in front of the body and shaking vigorously while phonating to facilitate jaw and tongue base release
3. Chest tapping to facilitate sensory awareness of tone placement

Block, in her article "Making a Case for Transmasculine Voice and Communication Training" [43], also advocates for focus on the jaw and base of the tongue. Utilizing imagery of a "ping pong ball in the back of the throat" or yawn-sigh with stimuli which include back vowels helps facilitate lowering of the jaw and tongue base for masculine-identified resonance.

Another perceptual target that research has shown may have a masculinizing effect on speech is /s/. Avery and Liss [27] describe masculine-identified voices as producing /s/ with a lower-frequency center. Giving the client perceptual cues (vertical, round) and describing a lower tongue position/rounded lips are possible facilitators:

1. Model a low-frequency vs high-frequency /s/ to the client, utilizing lip rounding with a lower tongue arch and lip spread with higher tongue arch, respectively.
2. Invite client to try both /s/ types, utilizing whichever cues (visual cues of vertical versus horizontal hand movements or tongue shifting, verbal cues) the client feels are helpful. Ask client to self-label the different /s/ productions and utilize their descriptors.
3. Additionally, pair with back vowels (/su/, /so/, /sɑ/, /sɔ/) to aid the client in creating and maintaining a more pharyngeal tone focus. Invite client to describe the placement and feeling of each sound.

When exploring resonance, it is important to normalize vocal play and production of abnormal, even unpleasant sounds. Encouraging the client to approach resonance with openness, curiosity, and without judging the sound can help make the process more comfortable as well as reduce extraneous thoughts that may interfere with discovering resonance that is more fitting of the client's desired gender expression. As in every facet of voice masculinization, client feedback should be sought continually to ensure the target voice quality is ideal and authentic to them.

Intonation, Pitch Variation, and Language

Investigation of the currently available literature reveals that more extensive falling intonation, and to a lesser extent, limited pitch variation, may be an effective treatment target for those wishing to "masculinize" their voice [27, 48, 52, 53]. The use of frequency tracing software may be a helpful visual cue to monitor falling intonation in real time and/or retrospectively. There exists frequency tracing software that will also provide information on pitch range within a recorded utterance, which can be used to give retrospective feedback to a client seeking to limit their pitch variability.

Based on client goals, assertive speech may be targeted alongside downward-sloping intonation. Assertive speech contains a greater number of declarative and imperative sentences, which lend themselves to falling intonation more readily than do exclamatory and interrogative sentences. Block [43] provides an example of modifying how to seek information in an occupational setting. For example, instead of the high affiliative "Can I ask you a question?," an assertive alternative is "Quick question." A suggested activity is to examine a scenario in which a client would like to portray assertiveness and to think of conversational topics which might arise. Together, client and clinician can explore the different ways in which one can express a thought on the spectrum of assertiveness and affiliation.

To provide additional examples, a work deadline can be expressed in several different ways:

Assertive: I need this done by Friday. (AS)
Affiliative: How do you feel about a deadline of Friday? (AF)
Affiliative/assertive: Let's work to get this done by Friday! (AFAS)
Neither: This should really get done by Friday.
[45] [54]

Respiration

Some transmasculine individuals elect to utilize chest binding techniques, often with bandages or constricting binders, which shapes chest contour and may provide relief from negative feelings about their appearance. There is evidence to support that binders can negatively impact respiration, a vital subsystem of voice production [12, 18, 55]. Clinicians should provide education regarding the possible effect of chest binding on respiration and voice, promote healthy usage of chest binding techniques, and work around any limitation which may arise by focusing on relaxation of the thorax and lower abdomen.

Generalization of Voice and Communication Techniques

Generalization, or the semi-conscious utilization of behaviors targeted in intervention into everyday situations, of the target voice is simultaneously the most difficult and most impactful aspect of voice training. Speech-language pathologists of all disciplines utilize a hierarchy of generalization which gradually increases in difficulty to ensure that clients receive adequate support to experience success. Below is a suggested hierarchy to follow when generalizing skills:

(a) Sound
(b) Word
(c) Phrase
(d) Sentence

(e) Functional phrases
(f) Paragraph
(g) Spontaneous sentence
(h) Multiple spontaneous sentences
(i) Monologue
(j) Conversation

Suggestions to support generalization:

1. Utilize material that is relevant to the client's interests and everyday activities to increase motivation, involvement, and effectiveness:

   (a) Functional phrases, defined as phrases that are within a client's daily vernacular ("Hi how's it going?" "What's up?" "What do you want for dinner?"), have been shown to be effective for generalizing [56]. These are most meaningful when produced by the client.

2. Move between levels as needed. Simply because the client has surpassed a level in a given session does not mean they will be able to replicate in practice or in the next session. Progress is not always linear.
3. It is a big step to shift from reading aloud to spontaneous speech. Cognitive load theory states that human brains have the capacity to process information. Human working memory is only able to hold a small amount of information at any one time, and instructional methods should avoid overload to maximize learning. Novel information and concepts require more attention and working memory and thereby have a heavy "cognitive load." This reduces the brain's capacity to process other information [57]. Spontaneous speech is posited to have a higher cognitive load than speech in reading, as the brain must synthesize many different processes to decide how to respond both conceptually and motorically. Consequently, if producing the target voice is not yet a familiar task, the high cognitive load will not allow for success at the conversational level. Effective therapy will allow the client adequate time to practice balancing that cognitive load.
4. When clients reach the conversational level, consider varying the topic (familiar or unfamiliar), context (group or individual) setting (familiar or unfamiliar, public or private), and communication partner (familiar or unfamiliar, same gender or other gender) [45] to adjust difficulty and increase the client's confidence.
5. Consider the level of emotional comfort your client is experiencing. When utilizing the voice in a novel manner, clients may express concerns about naturalness and being perceived as "putting on" a voice. This could be an indicator for a change in a previously agreed-upon treatment target or simply the result of anxiety with unfamiliarity of the new technique which may subside with time. Regardless, these concerns should be addressed thoughtfully and empathetically with the client before moving forward and throughout the voice work.
6. Utilize the principles of motor learning to increase efficacy of practice both in session and at home (see Table 11.1) [58, 59].

Table 11.1 Principles of motor learning (summarized)

Feature of practice	Choice	Supports learning of new skill	Supports retention of skill
Amount of trials	Small—Low number Large—High number	Small	Large
Practice distribution over time (equal number of trials)	Massed—Over a shorter period of time Spaced—Over a longer period of time	Massed	Spaced
Variability of targets in practice	Constant—Practice with the same target in same context Variable—Practice with different targets in different contexts	Constant	Variable
Practice schedule	Blocked—One target skill practiced at a time Random—Multiple target skills practiced at a time	Blocked	Random
Focus of attention	Internal—Focus on bodily movements External—Focus on effects of movements (e.g., sound)	Internal (though can be detrimental)	External
Type of feedback on performance	Knowledge of performance—Qualitative, target-specific Knowledge of accuracy—Correct/incorrect	Knowledge of performance	Knowledge of results
Frequency of feedback	Often Occasional	Often	Occasional
Timing of feedback	Immediate—Directly following trial Delayed—Time given after trial before feedback given	Immediate	Delayed

Maas et al. [58], Helding [59]

Additional Treatment Considerations

Gender-affirming voice and communication training is unique as it is this work which demonstrates results that are most influenced by perception distal or external to the client. Azul et al. [12] described gender perception as the "outcome of a collaborative 'doing' involving both speaker and listener(s) and the norms of sex and gender prevalent in different social and cultural settings." A listener's perception is substantially impacted by their life experiences, assumptions, and preconceived notions, and as such, clients do not have direct agency over how their voice is perceived [60]. Demonstrated by the highly variegated and at times conflicting evidence in the present literature, there is no definitive method of changing perception that is bound to influence listeners consistently. Consequently, the vocal situation (voice function, sociocultural positioning, and psychosocial well-being) of the client is exceedingly important to understand. Azul [1] advocated for treatment plans that address not only the individual's specific goals for gender presentation but also the individual's response to their dissatisfaction with instances of being perceived incorrectly or inauthentically. It is recommended that the treatment includes "developing and practicing strategies for responding confidently to instances of gender misattributions in everyday encounters." A model for effective treatment could include collaboration between the clinician and the client in examining the stressors (being misgendered on the phone, hearing voice recordings played back, lack of acceptance by family) and resources (supportive workplace, friendship, trusted psychotherapist, coping strategies). From there, a plan can be made to reduce stressors and increase resources where possible to provide an improved vocal situation and an increase in gender congruence and self-acceptance [11, 13].

Conclusion

There is a need for continued research into the vocal situations of transmasculine and TGNC individuals, as well as the effectiveness of voice masculinization training. Initially, testosterone to lower vocal pitch was thought to be the only treatment needed to achieve a masculine voice. Research has shown that this is an incomplete treatment for those wanting to masculinize their voice and communication styles. Current evidence is highly variable as to what constitutes a "masculine" voice, thereby only partially supporting the development of effective treatment protocols. The goal of voice masculinization is not always to be identified as male. Therefore, the definition of effective treatment is expanded to fit the needs of all individuals wishing to masculinize their voice. When developing treatment plans, clinicians and coaches alike should consider several important factors:

- Voice masculinization training is not exclusively for transgender men.
- Research into masculine communication is both limited and heterogeneous in its findings. Treatment targets must be client specific and client directed.
- Commonly held stereotypes about masculine communication were found to be incorrect or only partially true based on research. Clinicians cannot assume that clients agree or identify with specialists' personal ideas on masculinity.
- It is important to develop a collaborative relationship with the client, which includes understanding their gender expression and goals as well as the context in which they are living and expressing themselves.

Voice masculinization is a complex and nuanced topic which will benefit from further research and exploration. Ultimately, it is the job of the clinician to join the evidence available with a position of open mindedness and non-judgment to help clients achieve a voice and communication style that is congruent with their gender.

References

1. Azul D. Transmasculine people's vocal situations: a critical review of gender-related discourses and empirical data. Int J Lang Commun Disord. 2015;50(1):31–47. https://doi.org/10.1111/1460-6984.12121.
2. Van Borsel J, De Cuypere G, Rubens R, Destaerke B. Voice problems in female-to-male transsexuals. Int J Lang Commun Disord. 2000;35(3):427–42. https://doi.org/10.1080/136828200410672.
3. Watt SO, Tskhay KO, Rule NO. Masculine voices predict well-being in female-to-male transgender individuals. Arch Sex Behav. 2018;47(4):963–72. https://doi.org/10.1007/s10508-017-1095-1.
4. Irwig, M. S., Childs, K., & Hancock, A. B. (2017). Effects of testosterone on the transgender male voice. Andrology, 5(1), 107–112. https://doi.org/https://doi.org/10.1111/andr.12278
5. Damrose EJ. Quantifying the impact of androgen therapy on the female larynx. Auris Nasus Larynx. 2009;36:110–2.
6. Deuster D, Matulat P, Knief A, Zitzmann M, Rosslau K, Szukaj M, am Zehnhoff-Dinnesen, A., & Schmidt, C. M. Voice deepening under testosterone treatment in female-to-male gender dysphoric individuals. Eur Arch Oto-Rhino-Laryngol. 2016;273(4):959–65. https://doi.org/10.1007/s00405-015-3846-8.
7. Nygren U, Nordenskjöld A, Arver S, Södersten M. Effects on voice fundamental frequency and satisfaction with voice in trans men during testosterone treatment-A longitudinal study. J Voice. 2016;30(6):766.e23–34. https://doi.org/10.1016/j.jvoice.2015.10.016.
8. Cosyns M, Van Borsel J, Wierckx K, Dedecker D, Van de Peer F, Daelman T, T'Sjoen G. Voice in female-to-male transsexual persons after long-term androgen therapy. Laryngoscope. 2014;124(6):1409–14. https://doi.org/10.1002/lary.24480.
9. Van Borsel J, De Pot K, De Cuypere G. Voice and physical appearance in female-to-male transsexuals. J Voice. 2009;23(4):494–7. https://doi.org/10.1016/j.jvoice.2007.10.018.
10. Hancock AB, Childs KD, Irwig MS. Trans male voice in the first year of testosterone therapy: make no assumptions. J Speech Language Hearing Res (Online). 2017;60(9):2472–82, http://proxygw.wrlc.org/login?url=https://www.proquest.com/scholarly-journals/trans-male-voice-first-year-testosterone-therapy/docview/1948913172/se-2?accountid=11243. Accessed 17 Jan 2022.
11. Azul D, Hancock AB, Nygren U. Forces affecting voice function in gender diverse people assigned female at birth. J Voice. 2021;35(4):662.e15–34. https://doi.org/10.1016/j.jvoice.2020.01.001.
12. Azul D, Nygren U, Södersten M, Neuschaefer-Rube C. Transmasculine People's voice function: A review of the currently available evidence. Journal of voice : official journal of the Voice Foundation. 2017;31(2):261.e9–261.e23. https://doi.org/10.1016/j.jvoice.2016.05.005.
13. Chennupati, S. (2020). Communication assessment tool for gender-diverse people assigned female at birth. Master's thesis, George Washington University. GW ScholarSpace. https://scholarspace.library.gwu.edu/etd/dj52w555d
14. Leung Y, Oates J, Chan SP. Voice, articulation, and prosody contribute to listener perceptions of speaker gender: a systematic review and meta-analysis. J Speech Lang Hear Res. 2018;61(2):266–97. https://doi.org/10.1044/2017_JSLHR-S-17-0067.
15. Hardy T, Rieger JM, Wells K, Boliek CA. Acoustic predictors of gender attribution, masculinity-femininity, and vocal naturalness ratings amongst transgender and cisgender speakers. J Voice. 2020;34(2):300.e11–26. https://doi.org/10.1016/j.jvoice.2018.10.002.
16. Bishop J, Keating P. Perception of pitch location within a speaker's range: fundamental frequency, voice quality and speaker sex. J Acoust Soc Am. 2012;132(2):1100–12. https://doi.org/10.1121/1.4714351.
17. Gelfer MP, Bennett QE. Speaking fundamental frequency and vowel formant frequencies: effects on perception of gender. J Voice. 2013;27(5):556–66. https://doi.org/10.1016/j.jvoice.2012.11.008.

18. Block C, Papp VG, Adler R. Transmasculine voice and communication. In: Adler R, Hirsch S, Pickering J, editors. Voice and communication therapy for the transgender/gender diverse client: a comprehensive clinical guide. 3rd ed. Plural Publishing Inc.; 2019. p. 141–89.
19. Hudson AI, Holbrook A. A study of the reading fundamental vocal frequency of young black adults. J Speech Hear Res. 1981;24(2):197–200. https://doi.org/10.1044/jshr.2402.197.
20. Assmann PF, Nearey TM, Dembling S (2006). Effects of frequency shifts on perceived naturalness and gender information in speech. In Proceedings of the 9th international conference on spoken language processing (pp. 889–892). Pittsburgh.
21. Bachorowski JA, Owren MJ. Acoustic correlates of talker sex and individual talker identity are present in a short vowel segment produced in running speech. J Acoust Soc Am. 1999;106(2):1054–63.
22. Hillenbrand JM, Clark MJ. The role of fundamental frequency and formant frequencies in distinguishing the voices of men and women. Atten Percept Psychophys. 2009;71(5):1150–66.
23. Skuk VG, Schweinberger SR. Influences of fundamental frequency, formant frequencies, aperiodicity, and spectrum level on the perception of voice gender. J Speech Lang Hear Res. 2014;57(1):285–96. https://doi.org/10.1044/1092-4388(2013/12-0314).
24. Gelfer MP, Schofield KJ. Comparison of acoustic and perceptual measures of voice in male-to-female transsexuals perceived as female versus those perceived as male. J Voice. 2000;14(1):22–33.
25. Pisanski K, Rendall D. The prioritization of voice fundamental frequency or formants in listeners' assessments of speaker size, masculinity, and attractiveness. J Acoust Soc Am. 2011;129(4):2201–12. https://doi.org/10.1121/1.3552866.
26. Munson B. The acoustic correlates of perceived masculinity, perceived femininity, and perceived sexual orientation. Lang Speech. 2007;50(1):125–42. https://doi.org/10.1177/00238309070500010601.
27. Avery JD, Liss JM. Acoustic characteristics of less-masculine-sounding male speech. J Acoust Soc Am. 1996;99(6):3738–48. https://doi.org/10.1121/1.414970.
28. Booz JA, Ferguson SH. Perceived gender in clear and conversational speech. J Acoust Soc Am. 2016;139(4):2107. https://doi.org/10.1121/1.4950261.
29. Dacakis G, Oates J, Douglas J. Beyond voice: perceptions of gender in male-to-female transsexuals. Curr Opin Otolaryngol Head Neck Surg. 2012;20(3):165–70. https://doi.org/10.1097/MOO.0b013e3283530f85.
30. Bohn, Flege JE. The production of new and similar vowels by adult German learners of English. Stud Second Lang Acquis. 1992;14(2):131–58. https://doi.org/10.1017/S0272263100010792.
31. Flege JE. The production of "new" and "similar" phones in a foreign language: evidence for the effect of equivalence classification. J Phonetics. 1987;15(1):47–65. https://doi.org/10.1016/S0095-4470(19)30537-6.
32. Baken R, Orlikoff RF. Clinical measurement of speech and voice. 2nd ed. Singular Thomson Learning; 2000.
33. Holmberg EB, Oates J, Dacakis G, Grant C. Phonetograms, aerodynamic measurements, self-evaluations, and auditory perceptual ratings of maleto-female transsexual voice. J Voice. 2010;24(5):511–22. https://doi.org/10.1016/j.jvoice.2009.02.002.
34. Lakoff. Language and woman's place. Lang Soci. 1973;2(1):45–79. https://doi.org/10.1017/S0047404500000051.
35. Leaper C, Ayres MM. A meta-analytic review of gender variations in adults' language use: talkativeness, affiliative speech, and assertive speech. Personal Soc Psychol Rev. 2007;11(4):328–63. https://doi.org/10.1177/1088868307302221.
36. Carli L. Gender, language, and influence. J Pers Soc Psychol. 1990;59(5):941–51. https://doi.org/10.1037/0022-3514.59.5.941.
37. Palomares NA. Women are Sort of more tentative than men, Aren't they?: how men and women use tentative language differently, similarly, and Counterstereotypically as a function of gender salience. Commun Res. 2009;36(4):538–60. https://doi.org/10.1177/0093650209333034.

38. LaFrance M, Hecht MA, Levy Paluck E. The contingent smile: A meta-analysis of sex differences in smiling. Psychol Bull. 2003;129(2):305–34. https://doi.org/10.1037/0033-2909.129.2.305.
39. Boker SM, Theobald B-J, Mangini M, Ambadar Z, Cohn JF, Matthews I, Spies JR, Brick TR. Something in the way we move: motion dynamics, not perceived sex, influence head movements in conversation. J Exp Psychol Hum Percept Perform. 2011;37(3):874–91. https://doi.org/10.1037/a0021928.
40. Hess U, Adams R, Kleck R. Who may frown and who should smile? Dominance, affiliation, and the display of happiness and anger. Cognit Emot. 2005;19(4):515–36. https://doi.org/10.1080/02699930441000364.
41. McDuff D, Girard JM, Kaliouby R, et al. Large-scale observational evidence of cross-cultural differences in facial behavior. J Nonverbal Behav. 2016;41(1):1–19. https://doi.org/10.1007/s10919-016-0244-x.
42. McDuff D, Kodra E, Kaliouby RE, LaFrance M. A large-scale analysis of sex differences in facial expressions. PLoS One. 2017;12(4):e0173942. https://doi.org/10.1371/journal.pone.0173942.
43. Block C. Making a case for transmasculine voice and communication training. Perspectives of the ASHA Special Interest Groups SIG. 2017;3(1):33–41.
44. Davies S, Papp VG, Antoni C. Voice and communication change for gender nonconforming individuals: giving voice to the person inside. International J Transgenderism. 2015;16(3):117–59. https://doi.org/10.1080/15532739.2015.1075931.
45. Hancock AB, Siegfriedt L. Transforming voice and communication for transgender and gender-diverse people: an evidence-based process. Plural Publishing, Incorporated; 2019.
46. Davies S, Goldberg JM. Clinical aspects of transgender speech feminization and masculinization. Int J Transgenderism. 2006;9(3–4):167–96. https://doi.org/10.1300/J485v09n03_08.
47. Gelfer MP, Mordaunt M. Chapter 9: pitch and intonation. In: Adler R, Hirsch S, Mordaunt M, editors. Voice and communication therapy for the transgender/transsexual client: a comprehensive clinical guide. 3rd ed. Plural Publishing Inc.; 2012. p. 187–223.
48. Wolfe V, Ratusnik DL, Smith FH, Northrop G. Intonation and fundamental frequency in male-to-female transsexuals. J Speech Hear Disord. 1990;55(1):43–50. https://doi.org/10.1044/jshd.5501.43.
49. Hancock AB, Garabedian LM. Transgender voice and communication treatment: a retrospective chart review of 25 cases. Int J Lang Commun Disord. 2013;48(1):54–65. https://doi.org/10.1111/j.1460-6984.2012.00185.
50. François F. The effect of laryngeal manual therapy and laryngeal reposturing with voicing on fundamental frequency and estimated vocal tract length in transmasculine speakers. ProQuest Dissertations Publishing; 2021.
51. Mills M, Stoneham G. The voice book for trans and non-binary people: a practical guide to creating and sustaining authentic voice and communication. Jessica Kingsley Publishers; 2017.
52. Owen K, Hancock AB. The role of self- and listener perceptions of femininity in voice therapy. Int J Transgend. 2010;12(4):272–84. https://doi.org/10.1080/15532739.2010.550767.
53. Hancock A, Colton L, Douglas F. Intonation and gender perception: applications for transgender speakers. J Voice. 2014;28(2):203–9. https://doi.org/10.1016/j.jvoice.2013.08.009.
54. Wingate VS, Palomares NA. Gender issues in intergroup communication. Oxford Research Encyclopedia of Communication. 2017; https://doi.org/10.1093/acrefore/9780190228613.013.463.
55. Peitzmeier S, Gardner I, Weinand J, Corbet A, Acevedo K. Health impact of chest binding among transgender adults: a community-engaged, cross-sectional study. Cult Health Sex. 2017;19(1):64–75. https://doi.org/10.1080/13691058.2016.1191675.
56. Ramig L, Countryman S, O'Brien C, Hoehn M, Thompson L. Intensive speech treatment for patients with Parkinson's disease: short- and long-term comparison of two techniques. Neurology. 1996;47(6):1496–504. https://doi.org/10.1212/wnl.47.6.1496.
57. Sweller J, Nguyen F, Clark RC. Efficiency in learning: evidence-based guidelines to manage cognitive load. Wiley; 2011.

58. Maas E, Robin DA, Austermann Hula SN, Freedman SE, Wulf G, Ballard KJ, Schmidt RA. Principles of motor learning in treatment of motor speech disorders. Am J Speech Lang Pathol. 2008;17(3):277–98. https://doi.org/10.1044/1058-0360(2008/025).
59. Helding L. Voice science and vocal art, part two: motor learning theory. J Sing. 2008;64(4):417–28.
60. Azul D, Hancock AB. Who or what has the capacity to influence voice production? Development of a transdisciplinary theoretical approach to clinical practice addressing voice and the communication of speaker socio-cultural positioning. Int J Speech Lang Pathol. 2020;22(5):559–70.

Part III
Surgical Techniques to Aid Transition

Chapter 12
Surgical Concepts in Transgender Voice Change

Sarah K. Rapoport and Sarah K. Brown

A person's voice is uniquely tied to their identity. In fact, the voice communicates information about an individual's gender within the first 200 milliseconds of speech [1]. In this way, the human voice becomes a particularly important point of focus for transgender individuals. Attaining a voice congruent with one's gender identity is often a central component in the gender transition process. Vocal pitch serves as the most basic gender-specific voice characteristic as females generally have higher fundamental frequency (F0) than men.

Contrary to testosterone therapy in transgender men which deepens the vocal pitch, estrogens administered in adulthood and used by transgender women have no effect on the vocal folds or laryngeal structure. As a result, transgender women or gender non-conforming individuals seeking a more feminine voice maintain an anatomically male larynx despite the use of medical therapy [2]. Still, many transgender women and gender non-conforming individuals desire a naturally cis-feminine voice. Depending on a patient's goals and desires, elements of their desired voice change can be achieved through behavioral therapies, surgical procedures, or a combined approach involving both strategies. As discussed in earlier chapters, speech language pathologists work to address pragmatics, prosody, resonance and flow, and formant frequency in their therapy sessions with transgender women and gender non-conforming patients.

S. K. Rapoport (✉)
Department of Otolaryngology/Head & Neck Surgery, Washington DC Veterans Affairs Medical Center; Georgetown University Hospital, Washington, DC, USA
e-mail: Sarah.Rapoport@va.gov

S. K. Brown
Speech Pathologist and Singing Voice Specialist, SKB Voice Studio, New York, NY, USA

M. S. Courey et al. (eds.), *Voice and Communication in Transgender and Gender Diverse Individuals*, https://doi.org/10.1007/978-3-031-24632-6_12

In contrast, traditional voice therapies for transgender women have historically primarily addressed pitch. Yet pitch-based therapies have been shown to produce limited sustainable results even in cis-gendered patients, as opposed to resonance and flow-based therapies which have been shown by Katherine Verdolini and others to lead to sustainable and durable voice change [3]. We believe that targeting these characteristics of voice—namely, pragmatics, prosody, resonance and flow, and formant frequency—is at least as important to a listener in judging feminine or masculine qualities in voice as pitch alone.

Voice surgery, on the other hand, addresses pitch directly. Vocal pitch is understandably often a focus for voice change because elevated pitch is associated with a brighter sound and more feminine voice, which are important factors for patients seeking voice change with a feminine focus. Traditionally, surgery has not been recommended for transgender women. After all, surgeries such as the cricothyroid approximation as initially described and performed by Nobuhiko Isshiki did not allow for dynamic pitch change and postoperatively could be associated with increased vocal roughness. Over the years, several other procedures have been developed to accomplish pitch elevation which may not result in these same issues.

Surgical therapies for elevating vocal pitch depend on three fundamental principles: (1) increasing vocal fold tension, (2) decreasing vocal fold mass, and (3) shortening vocal fold length [4]. In the following chapters, we introduce the current surgical procedures performed to accomplish pitch elevation, and each surgery addresses these principles in different ways. The cricothyroid approximation (CTA) increases vocal fold tension, the laser-assisted voice adjustment (LAVA) and laser reduction glottoplasty (LRG) decrease vocal fold mass as well as possibly increase tension through scar formation, and the modified Wendler glottoplasty and feminization laryngoplasty decrease vocal fold length and likely increase tension.

Each chapter that follows is authored by a surgeon with robust personal clinical experience performing the chapter's respective surgery. Within each chapter, the surgeon addresses the preoperative assessment used to evaluate patients in the clinic prior to surgery, whether preoperative behavioral therapy is indicated and the role it may serve, the surgical technique, postoperative patient management, and expected outcomes including phases of postoperative healing and recovery, return to voice production, and durability of the procedure. In this way we hope that this surgical section of this textbook provides you, our reader, with a more thorough understanding of the current surgical techniques for pitch elevation.

References

1. Latinus M, Taylor MJ. Discriminating male and female voices: differentiating pitch and gender. Brain Topogr. 2012;25(2):194–204.
2. Schwarz K, Fontanari AMV, Schneider MA, et al. Laryngeal surgical treatment in transgender women: a systematic review and meta-analysis. Laryngoscope. 2017;127(11):2596–603.

3. Yiu EM, Lo MC, Barrett EA. A systematic review of resonant voice therapy. Int J Speech Lang Pathol. 2017;19(1):17–29.
4. Kim HT. A new conceptual approach for voice feminization: 12 years of experience. Laryngoscope. 2017;127(5):1102–8.

Chapter 13
Cricothyroid Approximation

Chadwan Al Yaghchi, Christella Antoni, and Guri Sandhu

Introduction

Cricothyroid approximation (CTA) was first described by Isshiki in 1983 [1]. The operation aims to increase the vocal pitch by stretching the vocal folds and increasing their tension by replicating the action of the cricothyroid muscle.

This chapter will discuss cricothyroid approximation and our modifications. We have modified the original procedure [2] by:

1. Increasing the tension of the vocal folds by subluxing the thyroid cartilage over the cricoid (Fig. 13.1). We achieved this by placing the sutures obliquely through the arch of the cricoid cartilage. The needle is inserted through the middle of the inferior border of the cricoid cartilage and exits at the anterior edge of the superior border (Fig. 13.2).
2. Drilling away 2–3 mm of the inferior border of the thyroid cartilage to increase the cricothyroid gap, allowing enhanced approximation, leading to further ten-

C. Al Yaghchi (✉) · G. Sandhu
Imperial College Healthcare NHS Trust,
London, UK
e-mail: chadwan.alyaghchi@nhs.net; guri.sandhu@nhs.net

C. Antoni
University College London, London, UK
e-mail: christella@christellaantoni.co.uk

M. S. Courey et al. (eds.), *Voice and Communication in Transgender and Gender Diverse Individuals*, https://doi.org/10.1007/978-3-031-24632-6_13

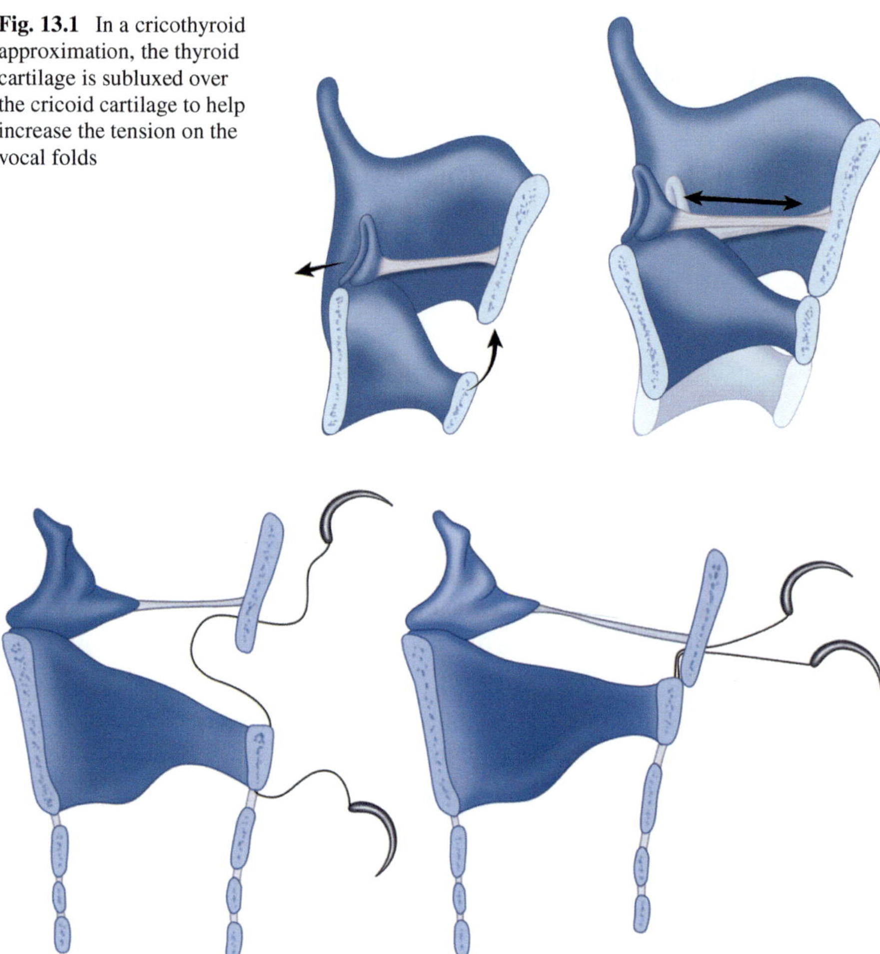

Fig. 13.1 In a cricothyroid approximation, the thyroid cartilage is subluxed over the cricoid cartilage to help increase the tension on the vocal folds

Fig. 13.2 Subluxation of the thyroid cartilage over the cricoid ring is achieved by placing sutures obliquely through the arch of the cricoid cartilage, as depicted here. The needle is inserted through the middle of the inferior border of the cricoid cartilage and exits at the anterior edge of the superior border

sioning of the vocal folds. This manoeuvre is particularly useful in individuals with a naturally short cricothyroid gap or a very low preoperative fundamental frequency.

Preoperative Assessment

A multidisciplinary approach to preoperative assessment, including a speech-language pathologist (SLP) and a laryngologist, is recommended when considering surgery for pitch elevation.

A full medical history needs to be taken, and questions need to be asked about the patient's perception of their own voice, their vocal needs and the impact of their voice on social and professional interactions. Reports of being misgendered repeatedly on the phone are a good guide to the severity of the problem. A history of previous dysphonia, laryngeal disease and laryngeal surgeries is particularly important. It is important to take into account professional voice use, such as lecturing, teaching and public speaking. Most forms of pitch-altering surgery will impact the vocal range or the quality of the singing voice, and this discussion needs to be part of the 'consent' process. Other factors affecting voice quality such as smoking, gastro-oesophageal reflux and use of corticosteroid inhalers need to be explored and documented.

Clinical evaluation should include stroboscopic examination of the larynx. This component of the exam is particularly relevant in patients who had a history of dysphonia or laryngeal surgery. Subjective and objective voice evaluation should be performed in every case. Perceptual voice evaluation using the overall dysphonia grade, roughness, breathiness, asthenia and strain (GRBAS) score [3] or the Consensus Auditory-Perceptual Evaluation—Voice (CAPE-V) scale [4] should be documented pre- and postoperatively. Fundamental frequency measurements should be documented in both free speech and reading standardised text such as The Rainbow Passage [5].

Patient-reported outcome measures (PROMs) are essential to deliver patient-centred care. The impact of surgical and non-surgical interventions to feminise the voice should be measured by the patients' quality-of-life improvement and sense of self rather than in hertz. In the authors' unpublished series, there was no statistically significant correlation between PROM scores and baseline fundamental frequency. We advocate the use of the ten-item voice handicap index (VHI-10) [6] and the Trans Women Voice Questionnaire (TWVQ) [7].

Role of Preoperative Therapy

When cricothyroid approximation is being considered, it is important to emphasise that surgery is only one aspect of the voice feminisation process and voice therapy plays a crucial role before and after surgery. Voice therapy in male-to-female gender transition has two aims: voice feminisation and the prevention and treatment of voice disorders.

The success of pitch elevation voice therapy and the longevity of the results vary in the literature. Dacakis reported in a cohort of ten patients a fundamental frequency increase between 10 and 78 Hz (mean 24.79 Hz). At presentation mean fundamental frequencies were 125.5 Hz, 168.1 Hz at discharge and 146.5 Hz at follow-up [8]. Soderpalm et al. reported reading fundamental frequencies of 138.8 Hz, 149.3 Hz and 157.3 Hz at first presentation, end of therapy and at long-term follow-up visit [9], while Gelfer and Tice results 123 Hz, 194 Hz and 155 Hz at the three time points [10]. In the authors' experience, voice feminisation therapy is very effective at elevating the pitch and associated with high patient satisfaction.

In fact only 20% of transgender patients referred to our institute are referred for voice feminisation surgery.

The second aim of preoperative voice therapy is to address voice disorders such as muscle tension dysphonia and laryngeal hyperfunction, the latter being a common pattern in untrained transgender voice due to inappropriate use of the larynx to achieve a feminine pitch. Kanagalingam et al. reported a high incidence of preoperative voice irregularity as an indicator of laryngeal hyperfunction. Surgery outcomes were better in those with lower voice irregularity and higher compliance with voice therapy [2]. Similarly, Yang et al. argued that speaking in an artificially elevated pitch can lead to a persistent state of tension in the vocal cords, akin to muscle tension dysphonia [11]. Preoperative voice therapy can identify and address these issues leading to better long-term outcomes.

Prior to cricothyroid approximation, an assessment by the SLP and surgeon is necessary. The SLP may primarily address postoperative voice care advice and objective voice measures of fundamental frequency. The surgeon will primarily address the benefits and limitations of surgery. It is helpful to inform clients that the lower notes of their voice are likely to be eliminated and that their voice will remain hoarse for between 2 and 4 weeks, with louder volume taking longer to build up after surgery. Together, the team sets the patient's expectations for postoperative results. Patients are seen initially at 2 weeks after surgery.

Although the authors' experience is that voice surgery outcomes tend to be enhanced and better sustained if the client has undergone a course of voice therapy first, some clients prefer to move to a surgical procedure quickly or without any SLP intervention. For those clients with no previous SLP input, it is recommended that basic exercises are covered at the-pre surgery assessment such as forward resonance exercises.

Surgical Technique

The procedure can be performed under local or general anaesthesia. Proponents of local anaesthesia argue that allowing the patient to vocalise during the surgery will enable the surgeon to adjust the approximation to achieve ideal pitch. However, in the authors' experience, early pitch following surgery is highly unstable and will drop with time. The 'ideal pitch' achieved on the operating table may not be maintained, and the aim of surgery should be to try to close the cricothyroid space.

Therefore, at our institution, cricothyroid approximation is performed under general anaesthesia in a supine position with the neck extended:

1. On induction, patients receive a dose of dexamethasone and a broad-spectrum antibiotic.

2. A 4-cm, transverse, skin incision is made within a natural skin crease between the thyroid and cricoid cartilages. Preoperative infiltration with 2% lignocaine + 1:80000 adrenaline solution is also routine.
3. Subplatysmal dissection is carried out superiorly and inferiorly. Dissection should be limited to the height of the larynx to minimise the surgical cavity and reduce the need for a surgical drain.
4. The strap muscles are divided in the midline and retracted laterally to expose the larynx.
5. Two horizontal mattress sutures, between the cricoid and the thyroid cartilage, are then placed on both sides of the midline using a double-ended 2.0 non-absorbable braided polyfilament suture (2.0 Ethibond) (Fig. 13.3). The sutures are placed extramucosally in the lower half of the thyroid cartilage below the level of the vocal folds. If the thyroid cartilage is ossified, holes are drilled using a 1.5-millimetre cutting burr. It is often necessary to remove the most medial part of the cricothyroid muscle using bipolar diathermy to fully expose the cricoid cartilage.
6. Note: Cricothyroid approximation can be combined with thyroid cartilage reduction and in such cases is performed at this stage of the procedure (Fig. 13.4).
7. Finally, we close our surgical wound. The strap muscles are then closed at the midline with their medial edges overlapping over the excised thyroid notch to mask any irregularity of the cartilage edge. Fascial tears should be closed, to cover the exposed strap muscle fibres, to reduce the risk of skin adherence to the muscle resulting in undesirable skin ‘puckering’ post-surgery. The platysma is closed with an absorbable suture, and the skin is closed using a subcuticular monofilament (4.0 Monocryl) and Steri-Strips. A suction drainage is very rarely required if the surgical technique is meticulous.

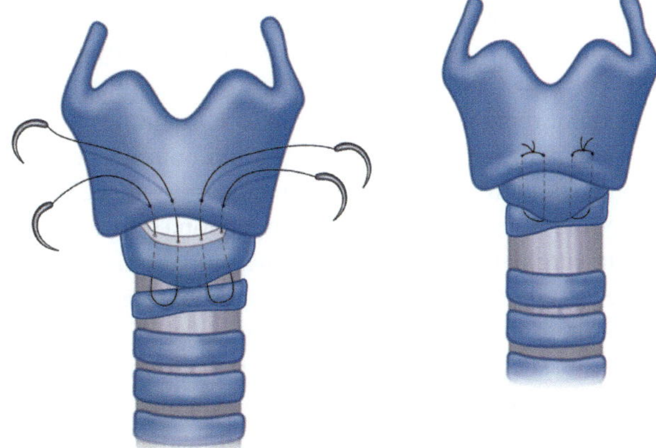

Fig. 13.3 Two horizontal mattress sutures are placed between the cricoid and the thyroid cartilage on either side of midline, as shown here

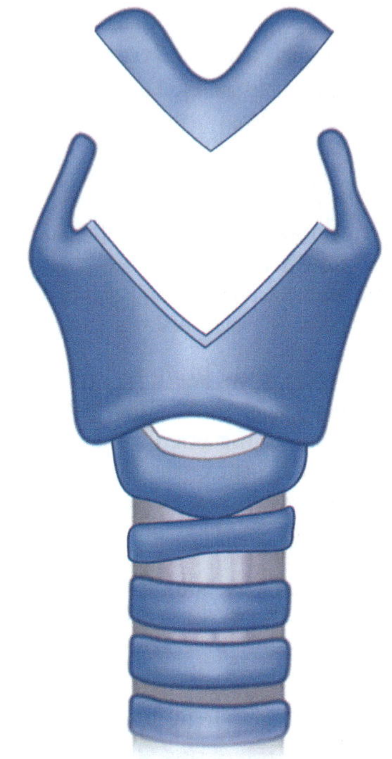

Fig. 13.4 Cricothyroid approximation can be combined with thyroid cartilage reduction, as demonstrated in this figure

Postoperative Management

The operation is performed as a same-day procedure, and the patient is discharged with appropriate analgesia and a 5-day course of a broad-spectrum antibiotic. If non-dissolvable sutures are used for skin closure, they need to be removed in 7 days.

Total voice rest is not required after cricothyroid approximation; however relative voice rest for a few days might be helpful to allow the patient to adapt to the tension of their vocal folds and reduce straining.

Postoperative voice therapy should commence 2 weeks after surgery. Therapy should start with general post-phonosurgery voice rehabilitation. Recovery after cricothyroid approximation varies with some patients experiencing initial dysphonia due to surgical oedema, tension and voice strain and pitch fluctuations. Initial voice therapy follow-up focuses on voice rehabilitation exercises and voice monitoring. Post-surgery recordings can be made as well as a basic programme of gentle voice exercises such as those involving nasal sounds /m/, /n/ and /ng/ and short glides. Once voice function has resumed to a greater degree, exercises can extend in length and variety. Some clients opt to continue on a voice therapy programme after pitch elevation surgery to maximise their voice presentation, enhance their vocal confidence and/or develop additional skills such as safe voice projection. Close working between ENT and SLP professionals ensures that voice outcomes are maximised for clients who seek our services.

Expected Outcomes

Cricothyroid approximation results in objective pitch elevation and high patient satisfaction. However, the results vary significantly across the published literature. Most published outcomes are small case series with no randomisation or control groups making data interpretation difficult.

In a systematic review, Van Damme et al. reported a wide range of pitch elevation ranging from 12 Hz to 108 Hz [12]. However, these two studies appear to be outliers, and the majority of the other studies included in the analysis reported an increase of fundamental frequency between 30 and 55 Hz. Similarly, Song and Jiang reported an average fundamental frequency increase of 44.97 Hz across seven studies that met the inclusion criteria of their meta-analysis [13]. In the authors' experience, a 71 Hz increase in free speech modal frequency and 74.7 Hz reading frequency were achieved at 2 weeks postoperatively, with subsequent drop at 6 months to 56.9 Hz and 51 Hz, respectively [2].

Long-term outcomes of cricothyroid approximation are rarely reported. Mora et al. showed a significant initial increase following cricothyroid approximation which deteriorated continuously up to 48 months follow-up. At 6 months postoperatively, the mean fundamental frequency increase was 42 Hz, dropping to 23 Hz at 12 months. This was in contrast to a glottoplasty technique, where pitch increase was maintained over time [14]. The drop in pitch appears to be related to a physiological adaptation of the vocal folds rather than loosening of sutures over time. Neumann and Welzel reported long-term drop in pitch in 22% of their cohort despite using metal wire sutures [15].

Pitch irregularity and dysphonia have been reported after cricothyroid approximation; however, the results in published studies appear inconsistent. Kanagalingam et al. reported a significant increase in pitch irregularity in the immediate postoperative period which improved with time and in those patients who complied with postoperative voice therapy [2]. Conversely, Mora et al. reported no change in perceptual voice analysis using the GRBAS score following cricothyroid approximation [14].

Postoperative complications are rare and often mild. In addition to general surgical complications such as bleeding, pain and infection, cricothyroid approximation can lead to procedure-specific complications. Poor scar or puckering of the skin, dysphagia, surgical emphysema and drop in pitch have been reported following surgery [13].

Notwithstanding its apparent shortcomings, cricothyroid approximation is associated with high patient satisfaction [12, 16] and significant improvement in quality-of-life measures. Mora et al. reported a drop in VHI-10 and perceived femininity VAS scores after the surgery [14]. It is to be noted that quality-of-life and PROM scores were inconsistently reported in the literature, making firm conclusions difficult.

Conclusion

Cricothyroid approximation is a safe and effective procedure for pitch elevation in male-to-female transgender individuals. The procedure is associated with high patient satisfaction and improved quality of life. However in modern laryngology practice, cricothyroid approximation has been largely replaced by Wendler's glottoplasty and its various modifications.

References

1. Isshiki N, Taira T, Tanabe M. Surgical alteration of the vocal pitch. J Otolaryngol. 1983;12(5):335–40.
2. Kanagalingam J, Georgalas C, Wood GR, Ahluwalia S, Sandhu G, Cheesman AD. Cricothyroid approximation and subluxation in 21 male-to-female transsexuals. Laryngoscope. 2005;115(4):611–8.
3. Hirano M. Clinical examination of voice. New York, NY: Springer-Verlag; 1981.
4. Kempster GB, Gerratt BR, Abbott KV, Barkmeier-Kraemer J, Hillman RE. Consensus auditory-perceptual evaluation of voice: development of a standardized clinical protocol. Am J Speech Lang Pathol. 2009;18:124–32.
5. Fairbanks, G. (1960). Voice and articulation drillbook, 2nd ed. New York: Harper & Row. pp124–139.
6. Rosen CA, Lee AS, Osborne J, Zullo T, Murry T. Development and validation of the voice handicap index-10. Laryngoscope. 2004 Sep;114(9):1549–56.
7. Dacakis G, Davies S, Oates J, Douglas J, Johnston J. Development and preliminary evaluation of the transsexual voice questionnaire for male-to-female transsexuals. J Voice. 2013;27(3):312–20.
8. Dacakis G. Long-term maintenance of fundamental frequency increases in male-to-female transsexuals. J Voice. 2000;14(4):549–56.
9. Soderpalm E, Larsson A, Almquist S. Evaluation of a consecutive group of transsexual individuals referred for vocal intervention in the west of Sweden. Logoped Phoniatr Vocol. 2004;29:18–30.
10. Gelfer MP, Tice RM. Perceptual and acoustic outcomes of voice therapy for male-to-female transgender individuals immediately after therapy and 15 months later. J Voice. 2013;27(3):335–47.
11. Yang CY, Palmer AD, Murray KD, Meltzer TR, Cohen JI. Cricothyroid approximation to elevate vocal pitch in male-to-female transsexuals: results of surgery. Ann Otol Rhinol Laryngol. 2002;111(6):477–85.
12. Van Damme S, Cosyns M, Deman S, Van den Eede Z, Van Borsel J. The effectiveness of pitch-raising surgery in male-to-female transsexuals: a systematic review. J Voice. 2017;31(2):244.e1–5.
13. Song TE, Jiang N. Transgender phonosurgery: a systematic review and meta-analysis. Otolaryngol Head Neck Surg. 2017;156(5):803–8.
14. Mora E, Cobeta I, Becerra A, Lucio MJ. Comparison of cricothyroid approximation and glottoplasty for surgical voice feminization in male-to-female transsexuals. Laryngoscope. 2018;128(9):2101–9.
15. Neumann K, Welzel C. The importance of the voice in male to female transsexualism. J Voice. 2004;18:153–67.
16. Matai V, Cheesman AD, Clarke PM. Cricothyroid approximation and thyroid chondroplasty: a patient survey. Otolaryngol Head Neck Surg. 2003;128(6):841–7.

Chapter 14
Laser-Assisted Voice Adjustment (LAVA)

Brian Nuyen and Lisa A. Orloff

Introduction

First introduced in 2006, laser-assisted voice adjustment (LAVA) was published by Orloff et al. [1] Previously, as a part of the original Wendler glottoplasty, the laser had been used to de-epithelialize the superior surface of the vocal folds in conjunction with endoscopic shortening. At its core, primary to the LAVA, the laser is used through the endoscope to vaporize the mucosa on the superior surface of the vocal folds away from the vibrating margin and thereby theorized to decrease vocal fold mass and increase stiffness through scar, enabling more rapid vibration of the vocal fold mucosa [1–5].

In silico and animal studies have more recently helped inform vocal feminization mechanisms. Titze et al. (2021) used computational simulation to explore anterior (Wendler) glottoplasty to examine how fundamental frequency varies with length of anterior glottis fixation, how glottic shortening can influence the sound pressure level (SPL), and the effect of fixing the ligament on fundamental frequency. They found that fundamental frequency increased dramatically when the anterior one-half vocal fold was fixed and that SPL decreased with fixation between the one-eighth and one-fourth mark. Inclusion of vocal ligament in fixation did not further increase fundamental frequency. Further, any fixation resulted in aperiodicity in acoustic

B. Nuyen
Department of Otolaryngology-Head and Neck Surgery, Stanford University School of Medicine, Stanford, CA, USA

L. A. Orloff (✉)
Division of Head and Neck Surgery, Department of Otolaryngology-Head and Neck Surgery, Stanford University School of Medicine, Stanford, CA, USA
e-mail: lorloff@stanford.edu

M. S. Courey et al. (eds.), *Voice and Communication in Transgender and Gender Diverse Individuals*, https://doi.org/10.1007/978-3-031-24632-6_14

signal. Titze et al. (2021) concluded that surgeons must navigate a compromise between pitch elevation and reduction in acoustic output power [6]. This elegant study demonstrates steady growth in our knowledge of vocal feminization since Tanabe et al. (1985) studied the effect of CO_2 laser vaporization in dogs. That historical investigation found such manipulation raised vocal pitch with resulting decrease in vocal fold mass and increase in stiffness from scarring in the canine model [2].

Preoperative Assessment

Upon establishment of rapport, key questions should be included in the history. It is important to understand the patient's goals and concerns for their vocal feminization, how they use their voice on a personal and professional basis, and what vocal tasks bother them both in general and specific to their gender-related communication and perception. Other related histories must be elicited as well—smoking/alcohol history, history of upper aerodigestive dysfunction outside of gender dysphoria, histories of voice-related trauma, and prior voice surgery.

Indications for LAVA continue to evolve as evidence emerges. In the original 2006 LAVA cohort, patient age ranged from 26 to 60 years, and no contraindications to this procedure appeared to arise for adults within this age group. In that study, the best results in terms of pitch of phonated comfortable /a/ were in those who had no prior history of phonosurgery nor of poor laryngeal hygiene (history of vocal abuse, smoking history). Patients who would like to avoid neck incision or an open approach may favor this scarless technique. As an outpatient technique that is relatively basic for most otolaryngologists/voice surgeons, this procedure additionally may be favored by patients for its ease, efficiency, and minimal general anesthetic time—typically less than an hour [1].

The use of LAVA is cautioned among patients who have had prior smoking history, prior history of vocal abuse, or uncontrolled gastroesophageal reflux disease. In the initial 2006 cohort, such factors were anecdotally related to postoperative decrease in pitch phonated comfortable /a/. Prior laryngeal trauma, head and neck cancer, laryngeal surgery, or history of overaggressive chondrolaryngoplasty that was complicated by anterior commissure detachment also should give the surgeon pause [1].

Physical exam should include a thorough head and neck exam and voice assessment, paying specific attention to the laryngeal framework. Furthermore, due to the nature of this transoral microlaryngeal procedure, it is essential to examine mouth opening, tongue size, loose teeth, and other anatomical predictors of difficult laryngeal exposure and perform lung examination. Preoperative laryngostroboscopy is a must, to bring attention to preoperative laryngeal anatomy including evidence of preoperative laryngeal pathology. To better objectively track patient outcomes for the surgeon and patient, we also strongly encourage providers to obtain standardized preoperative voice samples to save as a basis for postoperative comparison. The use of patient-reported outcome measures such as the Voice Handicap Index (VHI) or the Trans Woman Voice Questionnaire (TWVQ) also can help track subjective outcomes for improved patient satisfaction and surgeon quality improvement.

Role of Preoperative Voice Therapy

In general, voice training with a speech pathologist or vocal coach and surgery are prominent treatment options available for transfeminine vocal gender dysphoria. The combination of both approaches is complementary, yet many of these surgically inclined individuals emphasize that they desire an "automatically" feminine voice rather than simply an ability to "sound" feminine, as if they are acting, through behavioral voice change. While voice therapy can yield tremendous results with its particular behavioral attention to the diversity of vocal quality factors that feminize a voice [7], patients may still struggle with masculine voices that emerge with inadvertent phonation, such as with laughing, yawning, sneezing, and coughing [1, 7–9]. Many of the cohorts in the 2006 study had preoperative voice therapy and turned to LAVA for structural change that transcended behavioral effort [1]. Given that voice therapy has very little risk outside of cost, time, and effort and that vocal gender perception involves not only pitch and resonance but also formant tuning and phonatory pattern, voice therapy can certainly serve as a preoperative adjunct to LAVA.

Surgical Technique

Prior to surgery, multidisciplinary discussion of anesthetic plan and overall safety considerations with laser work in the operating room are important. Choice of airway management may be per patient factors and anesthesiologist and surgeon preference. In these authors' experiences, jet ventilation or high-flow humidified nasal oxygenation systems can be used. Alternatively, intubation with the smallest laser-safe endotracheal tube may be appropriate, but intubation may be associated with less than ideal access for microlaryngeal work. Furthermore, ascertaining compliance of the OR facility with laser safety is important as well. Laser system precautions include patient and operating staff eye protection, patient skin protection, plume hazards with appropriate smoke evacuation, and precautions related to fire hazards. Please see regulations as per Safe Use of Lasers in Health Care Facilities (ANSI Z 136.3) [10]:

1. After appropriate consent, the patient may be taken to the operating room and laid supine for general anesthetic induction. We prefer to rotate the operating table 180° from the anesthetist, place a dental guard, and use an appropriately configured laryngoscope, typically a Dedo laryngoscope for laryngeal exposure and associated suspension.
2. Using an operating telescope, high-definition examination of the larynx should be performed in detail, with photodocumentation. Special attention should be taken to document any laryngeal abnormality as well as the three-dimensional position and absolute and relative height of the vocal folds to each other, especially if there has been prior phonosurgery or laryngeal framework surgery.
3. After stable suspension and positioning, the operating microscope is brought into the field for optimal viewing of the vocal folds. It is important to see the

entire length of the vocal folds from anterior commissure to the arytenoids, ideally both folds at the same time.

4. A carbon dioxide laser is then set at 5.0 watts or less, usually around 4.0 watts and at continuous firing, in order to excise the tissue of the lateral portion of one of the true vocal folds along its entire length at a time. At this setting, excisional and coagulative hemostatic properties of the CO_2 laser are utilized. One of the hallmarks of the procedure is to diligently preserve at least a 1–2-mm margin of medial vocal fold as to not disturb the vibratory margin. The carbon dioxide laser is deployed with the settings aforementioned through mucosa and lamina propria, down to the level of the vocalis muscle. This technique is repeated on the contralateral vocal fold (Fig. 14.1).
5. After satisfactory completion of the procedure, we encourage using an operating telescope to capture in high-definition detail the immediate postoperative result for patient communication and education.

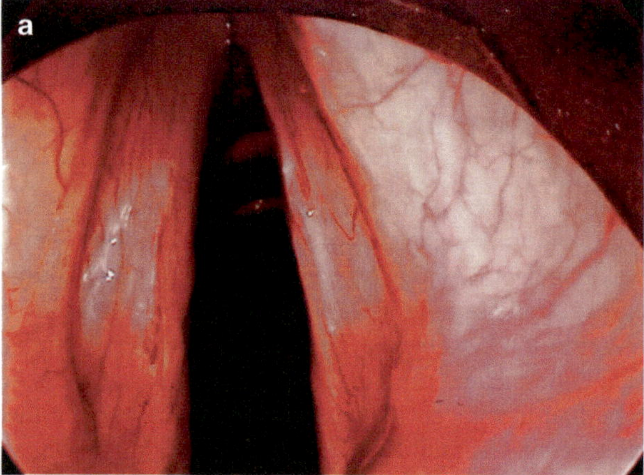

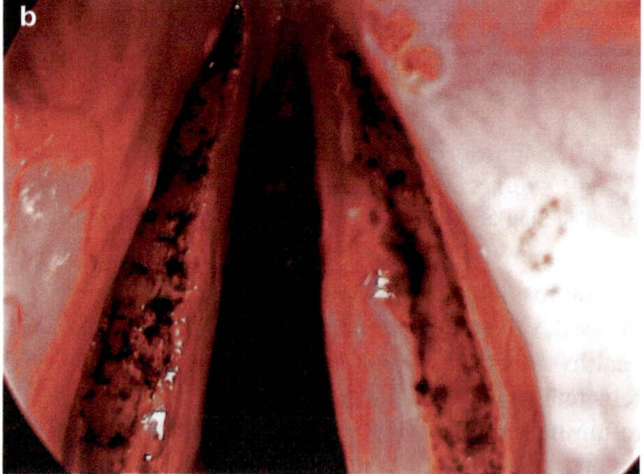

Fig. 14.1 Intraoperative photodocumentation of LAVA. (**a**) Photodocumentation of intraoperative microlaryngeal view of a transfeminine patient's larynx before LAVA. (**b**) Photodocumentation of intraoperative microlaryngeal view of the same transfeminine patient's larynx immediately after LAVA

6. Local anesthetic (usually 2% lidocaine) is applied to the surface of the vocal folds to prevent postoperative laryngospasm. The laryngoscope is then taken out of suspension and removed, and the lips and teeth should be examined. The patient is then turned back to the anesthetist for emergence from general anesthesia.

Postoperative Management

After the procedure, unless there are anesthetic concerns, the vast majority of these patients recover as same-day outpatients. We recommend 7 days of voice rest, with multimodal analgesia, with preference of acetaminophen and non-steroidal anti-inflammatory drugs over opiates. While every patient's pain experience can be different, postoperative opiate requirements are typically minimal or absent for the majority of patients. For most patients, regular diet is well-tolerated. For the first routine postoperative visit, we recommend seeing the patient in the clinic in 7–14 days after surgery for repeat laryngostroboscopy and additional counseling. Additional postoperative visits should occur at about 12 weeks or more frequently pending patient needs. By the 12-week mark, scar should be difficult to discern on postoperative in-clinic laryngoscopy. Granulation tissue if seen can be treated with anti-reflux medications and close interval follow-up.

Expected Outcomes

Healing Phase

Postoperative outcomes should start to approach their final form at around 12 weeks. In all patients examined in the 2006 study, stroboscopy revealed that glottic closure was preserved as were bilateral vocal fold mucosal waves. Although amplitude of mucosal waves appeared normal and symmetric, the gain in fundamental frequency was attributed to a decrease in tissue mass enabling a more rapid to-and-fro vibration of the vocal fold mucosa [1].

Return to Voice Production

In terms of postoperative expectations, in the original 2006 cohort that featured a group with considerable preoperative characteristic heterogeneity, the mean delta /a/ improvement was found to be 26 Hz. Of note, 78% of patients showed an average increase of 37 Hz in fundamental frequency with the range of perioperative change spanning −34 Hz to 58 Hz. Again, the patients with the greatest gain in this cohort were those who had neither history of prior phonosurgery nor of poor laryngeal hygiene. On average, satisfaction with postoperative voice and improved voice-image harmony predominated in the described 2006 cohort and can be mentioned as benefits associated with LAVA [1].

The postoperative VHI scores in the 2006 study represented an average handicap comparable to patients with Reinke's edema of the vocal folds. Patients who prioritize speech clarity and loudness as well as vocal range should be counseled appropriately, as these factors exhibited postoperative downtrends in the 2006 cohort. It is important to note that as demonstrated in this textbook, vocal feminization surgeries have their associated effects on the voice that transcend the primary goal of feminization. Unfortunately at time of this textbook publication, no meta-analytic comparisons regarding rates of defined complications across feminizing phonosurgeries have been performed, and there are tradeoffs with every procedure. Patients should thus be counseled appropriately regarding LAVA as an option in addition to other offered therapies [1].

Although pitch plays a major role in distinguishing male versus female voices, so many other vocal quality factors—such as breathiness, intonation, articulation, word choice, and inflection—are important in perception and communication. In 1990, Wolfe et al. concluded that there is "a narrow range separating the average fundamental frequencies of [transgender] voices perceived as male versus female" [11]. When fundamental frequency loses predominance as a clue to gender identity, other characteristics become more significant [11–13]. For some transfeminine women, the LAVA procedure may provide just enough rise in fundamental frequency through an increase in vocal fold tension, and decrease in vocal fold mass, for the postoperative voice to be perceived as female, especially if other speech characteristics are feminine.

Durability of Procedure

In the 2006 cohort, time to follow-up averaged 23 weeks and ranged from 10 to 72 weeks [1]. Given the lack of long-term follow-up, evidence-based conclusions regarding the durability of LAVA beyond a year are unavailable and are certainly an opportunity for further study.

It is important to note that definition of outcome success varies from patient to patient. Of note, in the 2006 study, three dissatisfied patients were consistently perceived as female by all five blinded third-party listeners. Appropriate perioperative counseling with open communicative strategies with patients will maintain suitable, patient-specific, and consistently transparent goals and expectations so that patient education, understanding, and treatment alliance are maintained [1].

Conclusion

Laser technology through endoscopic, microlaryngeal techniques can be a powerful, effective, surgically conservative, and safe tool to feminize the voice from a scarless perspective. Given the changes in vocal fold mass after vaporization, and that stiffness after healing would be expected to be permanent, LAVA surgery outcomes may be quite durable. Outcomes have been demonstrated to be favorable from standpoints of postoperative improvements in speaking fundamental frequency, patient satisfaction, and third-party perception of vocal femininity.

References

1. Orloff LA, Mann AP, Damrose JF, Goldman SN. Laser-assisted voice adjustment (LAVA) in [transfeminine individuals]. Laryngoscope. 2006;116:655–60.
2. Tanabe M, Haji T, Honjo I, Isshiki N. Surgical treatment for androphonia. Folia Phoniatr. 1985;37:15–21.
3. Koçak I, Akpinar ME, Cakir ZA, Dogan M, Bengisu S, Celikoyar MM. Laser reduction Glottoplasty for managing androphonia after failed cricothyroid approximation surgery. Voice. 2010;24(6):758–64.
4. Geneid A, Rihkanen H, Kinnari TJ. Long-term outcome of endoscopic shortening and stiffening of the vocal folds to raise the pitch. Eur Arch Otorhinolaryngol. 2015;272:3751–6.
5. Yilmaz T, Ozer F, Aydinli FE. Laser reduction glottoplasty for voice feminization: experience on 28 patients. Ann Otol Rhinol Laryngol. 2021;130:1057–63.
6. Titze IR, Palaparthi A, Mau T. Vocal tradeoffs in anterior glottoplasty for voice feminization. Laryngoscope. 2021;131:1081–7.
7. Nolan IT, Morrison SD, Arowojolu O, Crowe CS, Massie JP, Adler RK, Chaiet SR, Francis DO. The role of voice therapy and phonosurgery in transgender vocal feminization. J Craniofac Surg. 2019;30:1368–75.
8. Song TE, Jiang N. Transgender phonosurgery: a systematic review and meta-analysis. Otolaryngol Head Neck Surg. 2017;156:803–8.
9. Thomas JP, MacMillan C. Feminization laryngoplasty: assessment of surgical pitch elevation. Eur Arch Oto-Rhino-L. 2013;270:2695–700.
10. American National Standards Institute. For the safe use of lasers in educational institutions. ANSI Z. 2000;136:5.
11. Wolfe VI, Rutusnik DL, Smith FH, Northrop G. Intonation and fundamental frequency in [transfeminine individuals]. J Speech Hear Dis. 1990;55:43–50.
12. Kasyua H, Yoshida H. Chapter 3: Age-related changes in the human voice. In: Makiyama K, Hirano S, editors. Aging voice. Singapore: Springer Nature; 2017.
13. Coleman R. Male and female voice quality and its relationships to vowel formant frequencies. J Speech Hear Res. 1971;14:565–77.

Chapter 15
Laser Reduction Glottoplasty: Vocal Fold Reduction Surgery for Feminine Voice Quality in Transgender Women

İsmail Koçak and Okan Övünç

Introduction

Isshiki's classification of "thyroplasties" provided the first step of the surgical solution to voice feminization and revolutionized both the surgical field and the transgender population's expectations [1]. He developed and popularized the cricothyroid approximation (CTA) thyroplasty for pitch elevation and applied this technique to both cases of females with deep voices (i.e., androphonia) and male-to-female transgender cases [2]. CTA increases tension of the vocal folds by elongating the internodal distance, which results in a higher pitched voice (Fig. 15.1).

However, patients' satisfaction levels with this technique are not guaranteed. CTA achieved a postoperative vocal pitch above 180 Hz in only approximately one-third of patients, which suggested that modifying vocal fold tension would not suffice in most cases [2]. Furthermore, most of these patients were not transgender women, but women with androphonia. In another third of patients, the pitch was elevated but not to satisfactory levels, and in the last third, no change in pitch occurred. In the late postoperative period, stress relaxation resulted in a loss of gained pitch, usually from 6 to 18 months [3].

Due to these shortcomings of CTA, Isshiki attempted other additional techniques to remove vocal fold mass to elevate pitch. He performed CTA in combination with intracordal steroid injections, longitudinal incisions on the vocal folds, and vocalis muscle mass reduction. He also mentioned that lasers may be helpful; he used lasers to reduce mass, but only to a limited extent, and the resulting pitch levels were still not satisfactory. He explained that the evaporation of vocal folds was performed conservatively

İ. Koçak (✉)
DrVoice Clinic (Private Practise), Istanbul, Turkey
e-mail: ismail@drvoice.com

O. Övünç
Tekirdag State Hospital Otorhinolaryngology Department, Tekirdag, Turkey

M. S. Courey et al. (eds.), *Voice and Communication in Transgender and Gender Diverse Individuals*, https://doi.org/10.1007/978-3-031-24632-6_15

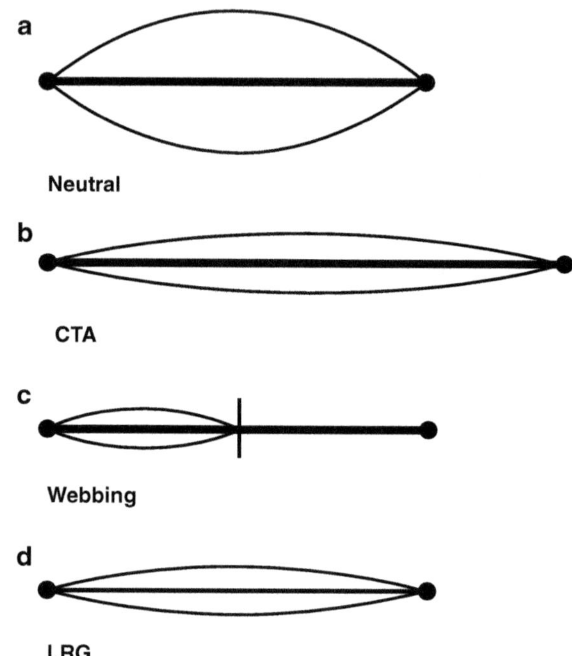

Fig. 15.1 Explanation of pitch-raising techniques by a string analogy. A string in a certain thickness and tension that can vibrate at a certain frequency is neutral (**a**). Raising fundamental oscillation by internodal tension, elongation, and thinning that resembles tuning an instrument is CTA (**b**). Shortening the internodal distance by adding another node and making one segment active and the other segment inactive like fingering a fret is webbing surgery (**c**). Fixed nodal distance and tension by thinning the string like changing thick string with a new thin one is LRG (**d**)

and remarked that this therapeutic modality seemed promising if adequate doses were established for laser reduction. These suggestions were the beginnings and constitute the fundamental principles of laser reduction glottoplasty surgery.

The senior author, Ismail Kocak, a laryngologist performing routine laser surgeries on vocal folds, designed and applied LRG to a transgender after failed CTA surgery instead of steroid injection, and the procedure was successful. The surgical video of this first case and voice outcomes are available on YouTube (https://youtu.be/0-ZNj4Hm5E0). After this case, the authors collected failed CTA cases and applied LRG. The results were highly satisfactory [4]. The high satisfaction levels were obtained especially in cases with FF values over 150 Hz and in younger patients (below 35 years of age). LRG provided an average of a 45-Hz increase in FF. Cases who reached above 180 Hz reported being greeted with female salutations in non-visual communications, such as telephone calls. Additionally, when compared with the results of successful CTA cases, the femininity levels were higher in the LRG cases.

Obtaining these results with LRG is logical, as the procedure reduces the layers that develop after puberty due to the androgen surge. Thus, LRG was used to treat non-transgender androphonic females and inappropriate androgen-induced masculine tones in children. Indeed, LRG became a primary choice for feminization and juvenilization of voice quality.

In the authors' routine practice, if the FF of transgender cases is over 150 Hz, LRG is preferred as a primary treatment option. If the FF is below 150 Hz, CTA is used first to elevate the pitch. A tracheal shave (which is actually incorrect terminology; "thyroid notch removal chondroplasty" is more appropriate) is performed during CTA if the patient prefers. After CTA, the patient waits for more than 6 months until CTA stabilization occurs and the process of stress relaxation is complete. Then, LRG is performed.

LRG is a technique that can be used primarily or adjunct to other surgical techniques that have failed to provide satisfactory results. LRG can also be used in women with androphonia, especially in constitutional cases and previous androgenic exposure (e.g., exposure in sporting women for increasing muscle tone and masculine body shape or for iatrogenic reasons).

Another advantage of LRG is that it is a same-day surgery. However, it risks vocal fold scarring and dysphonia. To prevent such complications, the surgeon must protect the free edge of the vocal folds [5]. Furthermore, vocal fold mass reduction levels should be appropriate. Mild breathiness could be a wanted result, as it resembles a sexy feminine tone. However, overreduction may result in glottic insufficiency, causing pathologic breathiness. In those cases, voice therapy may close the defect and the deformed cover layer.

LRG can be performed primarily or in a staged version, as follows:

1. *Primary LRG:* Feminine-sounding cases with low muscular tone are ideal for primary LRG. If FF frequency is over 150 Hz, then primary LRG should be considered for voice feminization.
2. *Staged LRG:* If the patient's FF is below 150 Hz, a staged procedure is more appropriate for achieving higher FF values. CTA (+/− chondroplasty) is performed first, and then LRG is performed after 6 months for better outcomes.
3. *Secondary LRG:* Failed CTA or webbing cases are candidates for LRG surgery. If expected FF values are not reached with CTA or webbing, LRG should be considered for secondary surgery.

Preoperative Assessment

Voice Assessment

Voice Analysis

The perception of femininity is significantly correlated with the mean FF of pitch [6, 7]. FF levels above 150 Hz provide more satisfactory results with LRG. In cases with lower frequencies, shifting to higher frequencies is usually possible with a staged/combined procedure with CTA.

Stroboscopy

Stroboscopy is performed to exclude any pathology prior to surgery. In some cases, Reinke's edema may be the reason for a deep voice. In this case, epithelium and superficial lamina propria (SLP) reduction would be the solution, rather than deep layer reduction. Furthermore, one-fourth of the general population may have sulcus vocalis and related lesions [8]. These are not a contraindication for surgery but may jeopardize the intact or smooth medial flap that is important for voice quality.

High-Speed Laryngoscopy and Digital Kymography

High open quotient (OQ) to closed quotient (CQ) ratios and speed quotient (SQ) levels are important in females compared to males [9]. Increased OQ and SQ values after surgeries may provide objective data about a shift from masculine to feminine vibration quality. Research should be performed to optimize this data.

Subjective Voice Evaluation

Subjective judgment is more crucial than objective data. Therefore, a simple visual analog scale of gender perception completed by multiple participants can be quite meaningful for optimizing the treatment process. Multiple participants listen to recorded voices and rate the perception of femininity, masculinity, and juvenility in the same recorded content on a scale from 0 to 5.

This technique is used in the authors' clinic. The patients rate their own voices and the responses they receive in their social environment. A dysphonia rating is also included in this visual analog scale for femininity, masculinity, and juvenility levels since surgical techniques may deteriorate the voice due to fibrosis and the healing processes.

Patient Selection

Patients are selected based on the following criteria:

- Age: Early age produces better outcomes. At ages over 35, satisfaction levels fall.
- Hormonal status: Anti-androgen therapy improves the outcome of surgery. The patients should be under strict control of anti-androgenic medications and have undergone testicular removal, which stops any androgenic effects. Any androgenic surge may result in a shift to masculinity.

Any previous transgender phonosurgery, such as CTA or endoscopic web formation, is not a contraindication for LRG. However, since this is a technique directly performed on the vocal folds, a risk of stiffness and dysphonia exists. Patients should be warned about this possible outcome.

Role of Preoperative Therapy

Preoperative therapy plays an important role in surgical success. If laryngopharyngeal reflux is present, voice assessment and analysis should be completed after treatment of the reflux. Additionally, possible cases of muscle tension dysphonia (MTD) should be diagnosed.

Voice placement and manner exercises are beneficial for creating realistic expectations. After surgery, patients may be less motivated to perform their exercises, and they may be prone to attribute any undesired effect, such as placement problems, to the surgical technique if they have not completed these exercises beforehand.

Surgical Technique

LRG surgery is performed under general anesthesia:

1. A rigid suspension laryngoscope is introduced, and the vocal folds are visualized under a microscope. Anesthesia is maintained with sevoflurane in a 40% oxygen/air mixture. A CO2 laser with a micromanipulator is used during the procedure.
2. The vocal folds are inspected bilaterally, palpated, and measured to evaluate any inhomogeneity or asymmetry before using the laser. The widths of both vocal folds are measured, and the lateral borders of their medial thirds are marked for incision. The medial third should be preserved for future vibration, as any violation or reduction of the medial third may result in stiffness and dysphonia.
3. The incisions are started at and lateral to the tips of the arytenoid vocal processes and extended along the vocal folds, parallel to the medial border. The epithelium and the SLP are reduced laterally by approximately 2–3 mm using a CO2 laser with a pulsed energy of 1–2 W.
4. When the cover layer (epithelium and SLP) is reduced, the power is increased to 2–3 W to reduce the intermediate and deep layers of the lamina propria.
5. After the vocalis muscle is reached, the vocal ligament is retracted medially to expose its lateral aspects and the muscle attachments. The vocal ligament is separated from the muscle fibers and is reduced by 1 mm from its lateral border with the laser.
6. Laser ablation is extended to the medial fibers of the vocalis muscle. The medial and posterior parts of the vocalis muscle are reduced by 2–4 mm in width and up to 5 mm in depth. The extent of ablation is tapered gradually toward the anterior-most point of the muscle, and care must be taken not to violate the anterior commissure or arytenoid perichondrium. The same procedure is repeated on the other vocal fold to complete the procedure. To prevent diplophonia, the final appearance of the folds should be mirror images of each other.
7. After this laser reduction procedure, both of the incised vocal folds are separated into medial and lateral flaps.
8. Three or more single interrupted 8.0 Vicryl sutures are placed between the lips of the incision sites and passed through the cover and the ligament with rounded needles, through both the intermediate and deep lamina propria layers. The medial lips are stretched and approximated to the lateral portion and then sutured in place (Fig. 15.2). These sutures stretch the medial vocal fold laterally and tense the vibrating portion between the conus elasticus and the lateral flap. This results in a thinned, lateralized medial vibratory portion of vocal folds and changes the shape of the vocal fold from rectangular to triangular, which is more typical of females.

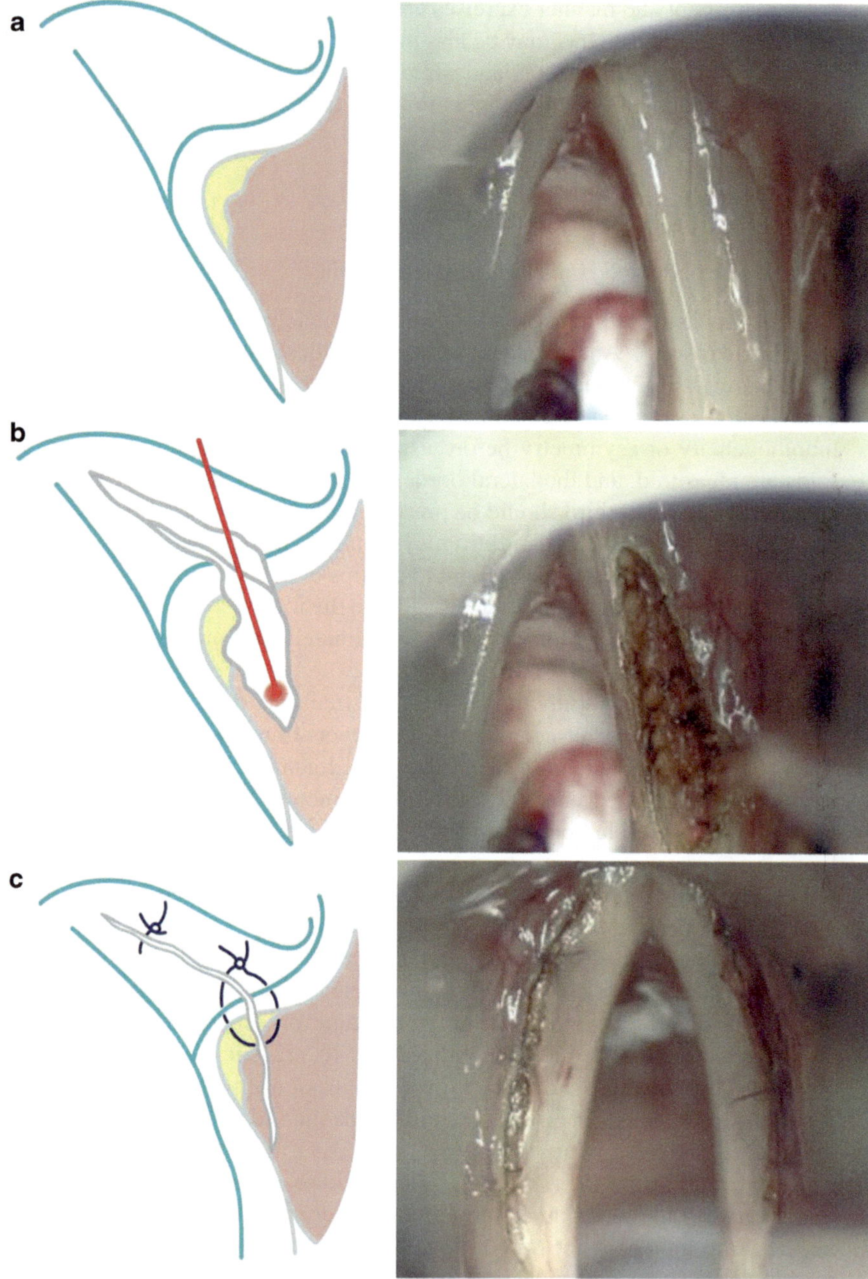

Fig. 15.2 Coronal section of the vocal fold and intraoperative view of the LRG (**a**). The cover layer, ligament, and the vocalis muscle are reduced longitudinally using the CO2 laser while preserving the medial vibrating portion (**b**). The medial portion is stretched laterally and approximated to the lateral portion and then stabilized with interrupted absorbable sutures (**c**)

The sutures are not to be removed. Suturing is essential not only for controlling fibrosis and healing but also for maintaining tension until the tissues heal, while the sutures are absorbed.

Postoperative Management

Patients are put on strict voice rest for 10 days until their first follow-up visit. This is followed by limited voice use that allows simple daily speech activities. High-performance vocal activities, such as singing or shouting, are allowed after 5 weeks. Late follow-ups begin after 6 months, at which point final outcomes can be assessed. In these follow-ups, the patients undergo a comprehensive evaluation of both the quality of their voice and the perceived results. In the authors' experience, the quality of voice continues to improve even after 1 year. Therefore, patients are called annually to observe their complaints and improvements.

Postoperative therapy is not mandatory if the patient achieves female tones and head projections; as mentioned previously, patients are hesitant to comply with a dedicated voice therapy schedule. However, annual visits determine whether problems are related to the patients' techniques, in which case intervention by therapy is possible. This includes brief sessions that involve singing therapy, placement techniques, and mannering.

Healing Phase

Postoperative vocal fold edema is usually observed until 5 weeks. The fibrin layer is observed at the incision sites, and the sutures are present. The patients are allowed to vocalize after 2 weeks, before which time they are advised to rest their voices. Laryngostroboscopic examination usually reveals reduced mobility of the mucosa and amplitudes, as well as inconsistent vibratory glottic closure with asymmetry and aperiodicity.

At the second visit at postoperative first month, the glottic edema resolves, and minimal glottic scarring is typical. Voice quality is mildly dysphonic, characterized by inconsistently short voice breaks and breathiness. Vocalization is produced with mild effort and some extralaryngeal tension. Almost complete glottic closure, with increased vibration amplitudes, mucosal waves, symmetry, and periodicity, is observed.

At the final, 12-month visit, all patients have good voice quality. The vocal folds appear normal with minimal scarring. Under stroboscopy, patients have complete, consistent glottic closure with periodic and symmetric vibrations. No hypokinesia or akinesia is observed (Fig. 15.3).

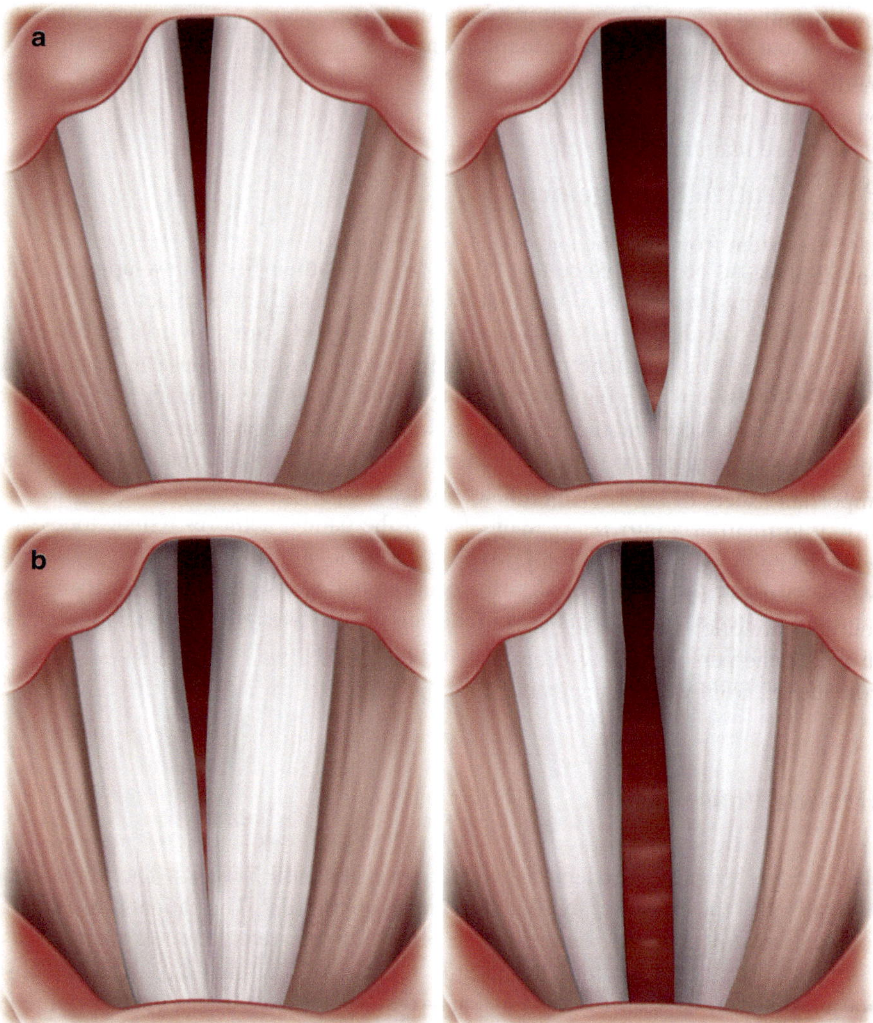

Fig. 15.3 Preoperative (**a**) and postoperative 8 months (**b**) stroboscopic view of same patient. Note the morphologic change in vocal folds. The folds are thinned with sharp margins. The maximum vibratory closed and opened views are same. No glottic incompetence is observed

Expected Outcomes

LRG increases the FF and femininity levels of voice, hence increasing the patient satisfaction. In our study first defining this procedure in 2010, FF increased significantly from a mean of 158.33 ± 12.14 Hz before LRG to a mean of 203.50 ± 13.34 Hz after LRG ($P < 0.05$) [4]. All patients achieved the expected pitch elevation in their voices. Four patients were completely satisfied with their voice outcomes. Perception of maleness (66.67%) reduced by a significant rise in perception of femaleness (85.00%) among total number of ratings ($P < 0.05$).

Long-term outcomes of LRG were investigated and found to be satisfactory. In a 2021 study by Yilmaz et al., LRG was performed as a primary procedure on 28 transgender women [5]. The pre- and post-surgery mean FF were 132 and 198 Hz, and the mean speaking FF were 123 and 194 Hz, respectively. A follow-up of 5 years or longer occurred for nine patients, and the comparison between the acoustic analysis results of the 1-year and 5-year follow-ups found no statistically significant difference. The pitch increment and voice outcome after LRG were found to be durable for at least 5 years.

LRG results in an FF gain similar to that of CTA. However, the FF gain after LRG is greater than that of other glottic volume-reducing techniques, including LAVA and intracordal steroid injections [10]. Furthermore, FF gain increases gradually over time with the resorption of edema and fibrosis at the laser incision sites. Therefore, a mechanical balance is established to counteract stress relaxation due to progressive fibrosis.

Like CTA, LRG has no effect on the acoustic tube, but reducing the bulk of the vocal muscle and ligaments shifts the vocal fold mass toward the female size range. Lateral stretching of the medial vocal fold tenses the vibrating portion between the conus elasticus and the sutures while thinning the cover layer, and it changes the shape of the vocal folds from rectangular to triangular, which is more typical of females. Therefore, LRG has the potential to compensate for the shortcomings of CTA both mechanically and morphologically without disrupting the previous CTA procedure.

Conclusions

LRG is primarily a feminizing surgery and secondarily a pitch-raising surgery. Its difference from other laser reduction techniques is that LRG is basically a glottoplasty procedure, because after laser reduction vocal folds are reconstructed with sutures. If LRG fails, CTA and/or endoscopic web formation could be added. However, LRG is less traumatic to the vocal folds compared to endoscopic web formation and less invasive than CTA. Furthermore, long-term results showed that pitch increment and voice outcomes of LRG are durable for as long as 5 years [5]. Therefore, LRG is the authors' preferred surgery for voice feminization procedures.

References

1. Isshiki N. Phonosurgery: theory and practice. Springer Science & Business Media; 1989.
2. Isshiki N, Taira T, Tanabe M. Surgical alteration of the vocal pitch. J Otolaryngol. 1983;12(5):335–40. http://www.ncbi.nlm.nih.gov/pubmed/6644864

3. Gross M. Pitch-raising surgery in male-to-female transsexuals. J Voice. 1999;13(2):246–50. https://doi.org/10.1016/S0892-1997(99)80028-9.
4. Koçak I, Akpınar ME, Çakır ZA, Doğan M, Bengisu S, Çelikoyar MM. Laser reduction Glottoplasty for managing Androphonia after failed cricothyroid approximation surgery. J Voice. 2010;24(6):758–64. https://doi.org/10.1016/j.jvoice.2009.06.004.
5. Yılmaz T, Özer F, Aydınlı FE. Laser reduction Glottoplasty for voice feminization: experience on 28 patients. Ann Otol Rhinol Laryngol. 2021:000348942199372. https://doi.org/10.1177/0003489421993728.
6. Coleman RO. A comparison of the contributions of two voice quality characteristics to the perception of maleness and femaleness in the voice. J Speech Hear Res. 1976;19(1):168–80. https://doi.org/10.1044/jshr.1901.168.
7. Van Borsel J, Van Eynde E, De Cuypere G, Bonte K. Feminine after cricothyroid approximation? J Voice. 2008;22(3):379–84. https://doi.org/10.1016/j.jvoice.2006.11.001.
8. Sunter AV, Yigit O, Huq GE, Alkan Z, Kocak I, Buyuk Y. Histopathological characteristics of sulcus vocalis. Otolaryngol Head Neck Surg. 2011;145(2):264–9. https://doi.org/10.1177/0194599811404639.
9. Tsutsumi M, Isotani S, Pimenta RA, et al. High-speed videolaryngoscopy: quantitative parameters of glottal area waveforms and high-speed kymography in healthy individuals. J Voice. 2017;31(3):282–90. https://doi.org/10.1016/j.jvoice.2016.09.026.
10. Orloff LA, Mann AP, Damrose JF, Goldman SN. Laser-assisted voice adjustment (LAVA) in transsexuals. Laryngoscope. 2006;116(4):655–60. https://doi.org/10.1097/01.mlg.0000205198.65797.59.

Chapter 16
Modified Wendler Glottoplasty: Endoscopic Bilateral Partial Cordectomy with Primary Closure

Sarah K. Rapoport and Mark S. Courey

Introduction

Wendler presented his endoscopic technique for formation of an anterior glottic web for pitch elevation in transgender women in 1990 in Salsomaggiore, Italy, to the Union of the European Phoniatricians. Although his original description of this procedure remains unpublished except as recorded in the proceedings of the meeting, several others have since published and discussed the technique [1–3]. The original Wendler glottoplasty was performed under general anesthesia through a rigid laryngoscope (Fig. 16.1—panel). The technique consisted of de-epithelialization of the anterior one-third of the membranous vocal folds with cold steel instruments taking special care to keep the vocal ligament intact. The defect was then sutured together to form an anterior glottic web using two Vicryl sutures placed along the anterior glottic defect to realign the de-epithelialized portions of the membranous vocal folds. To reinforce the suture line, fibrin glue was applied to the sutures over the glottic defect. Lastly, vaporization of the upper surfaces of the vocal folds 1–2 mm from the free edge of the membranous fold was performed with a laser, extending from the vocal process to the anterior commissure.

S. K. Rapoport (✉)
Department of Otolaryngology/Head & Neck Surgery, Washington DC Veterans Affairs Medical Center, Georgetown University Hospital, Washington, DC, USA
e-mail: Sarah.Rapoport@va.gov

M. S. Courey
Department of Otolaryngology Head and Neck Surgery, Division of Laryngology, Mount Sinai Health System, New York, NY, USA
e-mail: Mark.courey@mountsinai.org

M. S. Courey et al. (eds.), *Voice and Communication in Transgender and Gender Diverse Individuals*, https://doi.org/10.1007/978-3-031-24632-6_16

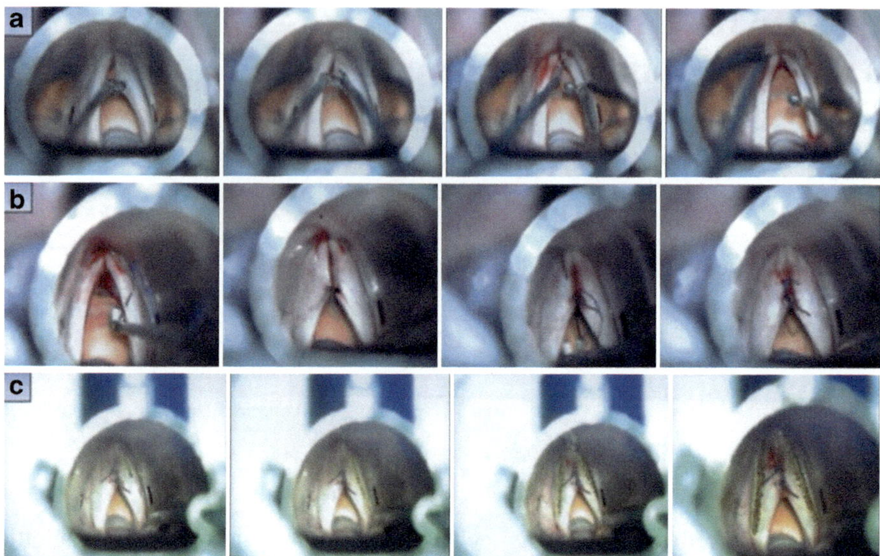

Fig. 16.1 Steps of the original Wendler glottoplasty procedure, adapted from Casado et al.'s surgical photographs

Increase in vocal pitch was obtained by decreasing vocal fold mass, shortening the length of the vibratory surface of the vocal folds, and/or increasing the vocal fold tension through scarification with the laser.

Our procedure is similar to Wendler's original technique of endoscopic bilateral partial cordectomy with primary closure; however, we have modified it in several ways. We therefore refer to it as the modified Wendler glottoplasty. We have altered it by (1) decreasing vocal fold mass by incising the membranous vocal fold along 40–50% of its superior and inferior lips or masses and then removing most of the vocal ligament from its medial surface; (2) generating a 40–50% anterior glottic web by placing one pair of Vicryl sutures at the midpoint of the vocal fold defect and a second pair within the undisturbed vocal fold tissue at the posterior aspects of the extension of our mucosal incision; and (3) increasing the tension applied to the vocal folds by stretching the superior mass/lip region of the vocal fold to the inferior arcuate line when placing our sutures to reapproximate the vocal fold.

The goals of defect creation are to remove tissue symmetrically from the upper mass to the lower mass or inferior arcuate line. By reducing the thickness of the ligament, it allows us to pull the upper mass down to the lower mass with our sutures. This effectively results in increased tension without the need to de-epithelialize the superior surface and rely on secondary healing. The goals of our suture placement are to increase the tension on the upper lip or mass region by pulling it to the inferior arcuate line and to close mucosa to mucosa at the posterior aspect of the defect. This maneuver reduces the risk of granulation tissue formation and creates a sharp neo-anterior commissure with intact vibratory tissue. Modifying the vocal fold in these ways elevates vibratory frequencies and allows us to maximally recreate symmetry to decrease the risk of postoperative noise in the fundamental signal that could be perceived as roughness and breathiness.

There are several notable advantages to performing an endoscopic glottoplasty for pitch elevation. Namely, its minimally invasive, endoscopic surgical approach enables it to be performed as a same-day, outpatient surgery. Additionally, ongoing studies continue to underscore the long-term durability of the surgery in sustaining pitch elevation as far out as 24 months after surgery.

Specific advantages to our modified Wendler glottoplasty include reliable elevation of pitch and improved quality of life in transgender women. Studies examining the outcomes of the modified Wendler glottoplasty have revealed there is a low risk of worsening voice quality after the procedure, and while this surgery should be pursued with caution in performance voice users given the variable loss of pitch range, we are noting patients who were singers preoperatively have been able to continue singing after recovering from surgery.

Important considerations, and possible drawbacks, when performing the modified Wendler glottoplasty include the relative fragility of the newly formed anterior glottic web. Patients often seek surgery for voice feminization during a period of transition when they may be planning to undergo additional gender-affirming surgeries. Enforcing that patients refrain from undergoing additional elective surgeries for at least 2 months after undergoing a modified Wendler glottoplasty is a critical part of preoperative counseling. In such cases that patients do undergo subsequent gender-affirming surgeries after modified Wendler glottoplasty, counseling the patient and their anesthesiologist to intubate the patient with a small endotracheal tube such as a 6.0 Mallinckrodt cuffed endotracheal tube with GlideScope intubation is advisable to reduce the likelihood of intubation trauma and preserve the integrity to the glottic web.

Preoperative Assessment

We recommend that candidacy for modified Wendler glottoplasty be established through a team discussion. As an example, we determine candidacy through an interdisciplinary, team-based conversation together with the patient, the laryngologist, and the speech-language pathologist (SLP). We offer all patients initially presenting to our practice seeking to make their voice more feminine the options for both surgery and voice therapy. We recommend strongly to patients that they pursue voice therapy prior to considering surgery; however, we do not consider voice therapy a requirement or prerequisite to surgical intervention. Our team considers factors such as potential for further progress in voice therapy and whether the patient's goals are congruent with the known benefits of surgery. The final decision to pursue modified Wendler glottoplasty is ultimately up to the patient.

When considering whether a transgender woman seeking to make her voice more feminine is likely to attain her desired voice with modified Wendler glottoplasty, it is helpful to tease out the patient's reasons for dissatisfaction with their voice. As previously stated, feminization of voice is achieved through (1) targeting flow, resonance, and pragmatics and (2) pitch elevation. As we have said, surgery only targets pitch. Many transgender patients are satisfied with pragmatic changes alone.

A common complaint among transgender patients is that they are unable to sustain elevated pitch and changes in their pragmatics in moments of expressing genuine emotion such as surprise, anger or during heated conversations, and in moments of intimacy. The emotional burden of feeling or being misgendered in these moments has been described to our team as causing disappointment, shame or embarrassment, and a feeling of disconnect between how one's identity is portrayed externally with how one identifies internally. In such cases where patients are able to sustain pitch elevation in routine conversation but not in moments of heightened emotion, modified Wendler glottoplasty provides an excellent solution for enabling sustained pitch elevation.

Role of Preoperative Therapy: Is it Indicated? Is there a Role?

The goals of preoperative voice therapy in transgender patients seeking voice change are to achieve laryngeal relaxation and efficient respiratory patterns. We target resonance, formant structure, feminine speaking patterns, and vocal efficiency. This results in a perception of increased pitch because of the forward placement of airflow during phonation. Voice therapy can be a noteworthy adjunct to successful voice feminization in patients seeking pitch elevation with modified Wendler glottoplasty [4]. In fact, we have observed that when patients learn to reduce laryngeal tension and strain prior to surgery, they demonstrate improved resonant voice use postoperatively.

Patients presenting to our voice center seeking voice change tend to approach their process for voice change in one of three ways:

1. The first group presents seeking surgery alone for pitch elevation. We encourage these patients to undergo one to three sessions of voice therapy while awaiting their surgery date to learn to reduce extralaryngeal tension and target oral and nasal resonance with improved vocal efficiency.
2. The second group of patients expresses hesitancy to undergo surgery and presents requesting voice therapy alone. Since the purpose of surgery is pitch elevation, many patients are satisfied with the changes produced reliably through therapy. In such cases, we intentionally revisit the patient's progress and whether therapy alone provides them with the voice changes they seek. The SLP may spend additional time trying to adjust pitch after changes in resonance, efficiency, and pragmatics have been achieved.

3. The third group of patients is eager for surgery at their initial presentation to our clinic yet understands the importance of flow, relaxation, and prosody in gender characteristics of voice. With these patients we usually work together to facilitate voice therapy and surgery for voice change.

We consider a meaningful course of voice therapy to be at least three to four sessions with a trained SLP. This recommendation was initially informed by literature advising that meaningful change in voice can occur through an average of 3.6 sessions of voice therapy [5]. For patients seeking sustainable voice change, three to four sessions of voice therapy is unlikely enough to achieve a feminine voice at the conversational level. Yet in our anecdotal clinical experience, many patients can produce their target feminine voice at the sentence level within three sessions [4].

Surgical Technique

1. Have anesthesia intubate patients with a small (5.0 to 6.0) laser-safe endotracheal tube and administer a single, high dose (10 mg) of dexamethasone steroid. Note: Preoperative antibiotics are not routinely administered for this clean-contaminated procedure.
2. Use a laryngoscope to expose the glottis completely from the anterior commissure to the vocal processes. Ensuring that this view is maintained after the laryngoscope is suspended is paramount as it enables accurate measurement of the length of the vocal fold (Fig. 16.2). Measure the length of the vocal fold to determine how much of the anterior vocal fold you must incise to create a 40% glottic web. If available, use the pattern generator attachment (AcuBlade™, Lumenis, San Jose, CA) with your CO_2 laser aiming beam to measure the length of the membranous vocal fold from vocal process to anterior commissure. Calculate 40% of that length to determine the length of your anterior glottic web.
3. Use the CO_2 laser, or cold steel instruments, to incise the bilateral medial margins of the anterior 40% of the membranous vocal fold along the fold's upper lip.

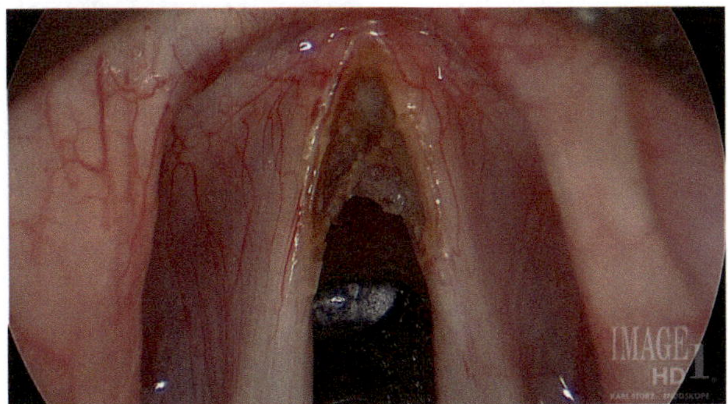

Fig. 16.2 Endoscopic view of the full-length vocal folds

Note: This surgery can be successfully performed using cold steel instruments. We find it advantageous to use the CO_2 laser with a pattern generator and will describe that technique here.

4. Use a microflap elevator to deepen your incisions anteriorly and posteriorly along the medial edge of the vocal ligament. Ensure that your dissection continues to the inferior arcuate line of the vocal fold. The dissection can be done bluntly or sharply or with a CO_2 laser.
5. Create a flap of mucosa and ligament at the inferior arcuate line (Figs. 16.3 and 16.4).
6. Use the CO_2 laser to excise or ablate excess tissue along this mucosal flap.
7. Suture the bare medial surface of the membranous vocal fold together. Here it is important to bring the upper margins together symmetrically and to have your suture incorporate the inferior arcuate line to help increase tension. We use four 4-0 Vicryl sutures on RB-1 needles. We straighten the needle from a half-circle to a quarter-circle. By placing the sutures through the vocal fold from top to bottom, two at the midpoint and two just posterior to the mucosal defects, we are

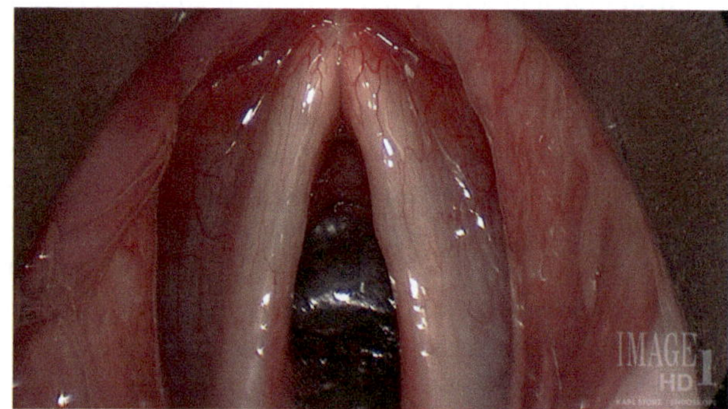

Fig. 16.3 Endoscopic view of the vocal folds using a zero-degree telescope illustrating the anterior glottic defect along the anterior 40% of the vocal folds

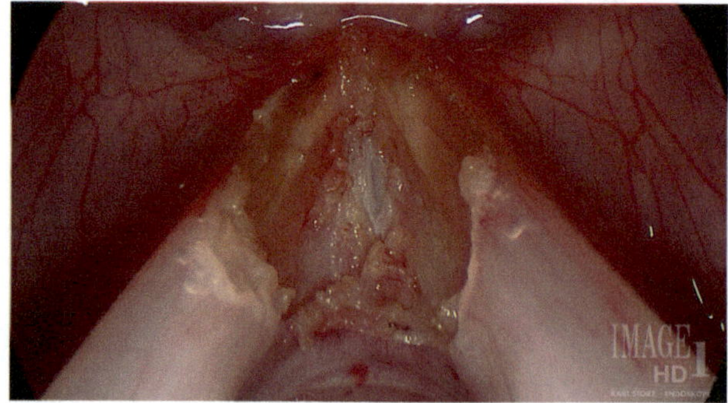

Fig. 16.4 Endoscopic view of the vocal folds using a 70-degree telescope illustrating the anterior glottic defect along the anterior 40% of the vocal folds. Note how the inferior mucosal flap is at the level of the inferior arcuate line

able to create symmetry during closure (Fig. 16.5). Other surgeons are able to throw a single suture from top to bottom and then bottom to top eliminating the need for the inferior knot on each suture. Regardless of preferred suturing technique, take great care to ensure your needles are placed symmetrically along bilateral vocal folds as the symmetry of your needle placement and bites of tissue ensures that the upper and lower vocal fold masses will align when the sutures are tied. Placement of the posterior sutures posterior to the mucosal defect will help prevent formation of neo-commissure granulomas which can lead to blunting of the neo-commissure and subsequent vocal roughness and breathiness.

8. Tie your sutures. The inferior suture ends are tied, and the knots are passed below the plane of the vocal fold by pulling and releasing on the superior suture ends until the knot is laid taut at the level of the glottis. It is critical that this tie be made with square knots; otherwise the knots will slip and likely unravel in the perioperative period. The superior suture ends are then tied to approximate the vocal folds in the midline (Fig. 16.6). The final goal is for the sutures to reapproximate the upper and lower lips of the vocal fold to mirror their original anatomic levels (Figs. 16.7 and 16.8).

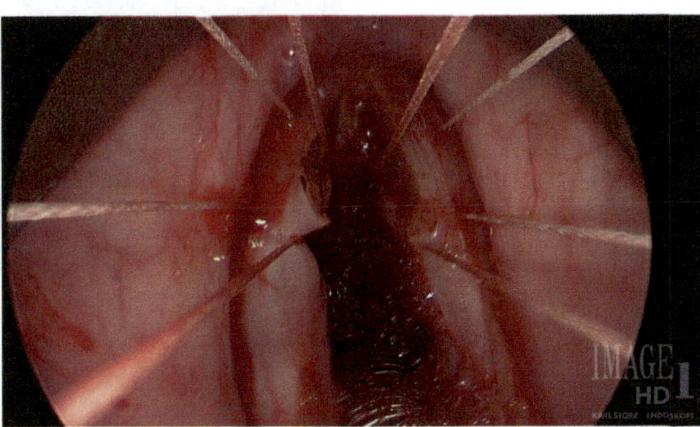

Fig. 16.5 Aerial view of the suture placements

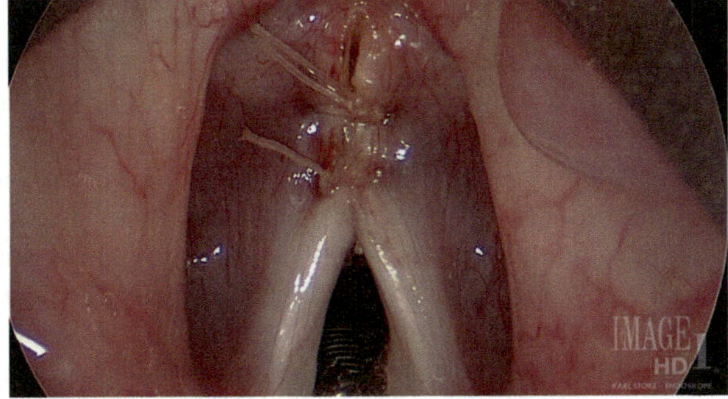

Fig. 16.6 Endoscopic view of the vocal folds with sutures in place

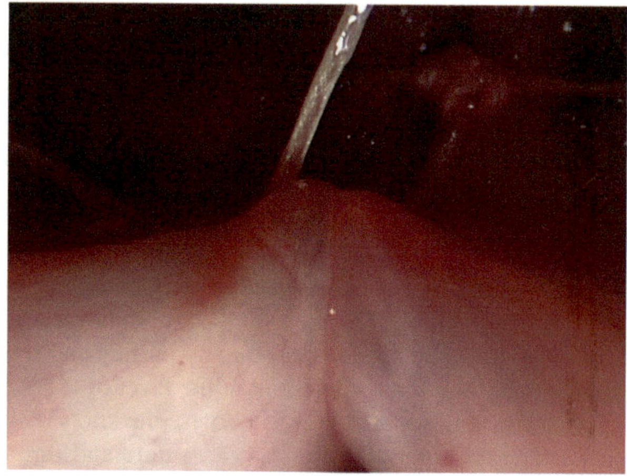

Fig. 16.7 Endoscopic view of the upper and lower lips of the vocal folds using a 70-degree angled telescope after the superior and posterior sutures have been placed to form the neo-anterior glottic web

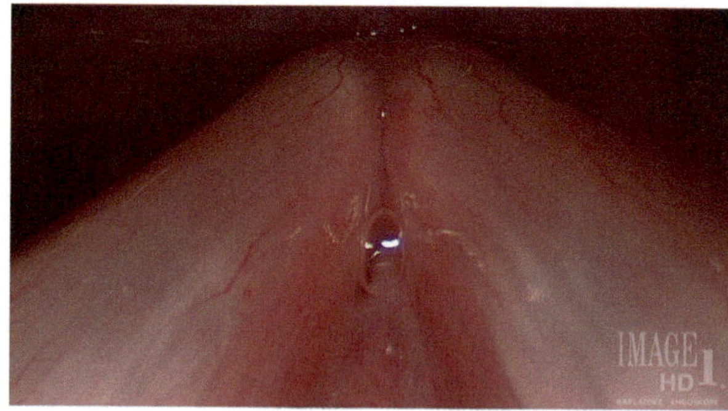

Fig. 16.8 Endoscopic view of the upper and lower lips of the vocal folds using a 70-degree angled telescope prior to beginning the modified Wendler glottoplasty. Note how the symmetry of these levels were maintained when the glottoplasty sutures were placed as demonstrated in Fig. 16.6

Postoperative Management

Patients are discharged home on the day of surgery after recovery from general anesthesia in the post-anesthesia care unit. Patients are asked to observe 1 week of complete voice rest to reduce risk of suture line dehiscence and vocal fold edema. For this same reason, persistent coughing or throat clearing should be avoided. Postoperative antibiotics and steroids are not routinely indicated.

Patients are seen 1 week postoperatively in the clinic, at which point indirect laryngoscopy is performed to confirm that the suture lines have remained intact and that the primary closure at the neo-commissure is healing appropriately. Patients who are compliant with voice rest and have not been excessively clearing their throat rarely show any evidence of significant edema or suture dehiscence. When patients are unable to relax their larynx in the immediate postoperative period and are continually clearing their throat or coughing, or do not observe voice rest, there is often marked edema and erythema edema of the larynx, but the sutures are still rarely disrupted.

After this initial postoperative visit, patients may resume efficient voice use for short periods avoiding vocal fatigue. Depending on each patient's ability to phonate efficiently with flow and relaxed laryngeal posture, voice use is advanced. Patients require an average of two sessions of semi-occluded vocal tract (SOVT) therapy postoperatively to aid in achieving this goal. By 1 month postoperatively, most patients have gained a usable conversational voice and have returned to regular voice use in quiet environments. Voice use is gradually liberalized over the next 2 months.

Expected Outcome: Healing Phase, Return to Voice Production, and Durability of the Procedure

Healing Phase

Mild to moderate erythema and edema of the vocal folds are typical at 1 week postoperatively. Despite the erythema and edema, a mucosal wave may still be observed on videostroboscopy at the 1-week postoperative visit. Crusting or scabbing along the suture lines is not uncommon and is noted to resolve by 2 months after surgery. Granulomas can form at the suture line and at the anterior neo-commissure. Granulomas on the superior aspect of the vocal fold along the suture line are usually of no consequence. When they form in the neo-anterior commissure, however, they disrupt vibration and anterior glottic closure. For this reason, we remain meticulous when placing the posterior suture to achieve precise mucosal reapproximation at the neo-anterior commissure.

Return to Voice Production

It is not uncommon for patients to experience a short duration of aphonia after surgery. The two main reasons for aphonia postoperatively are marked mucosal edema and erythema and increased extralaryngeal tension either from a lack of ability or emotional hesitancy regarding voice change. The latter is particularly common in patients who chose to undergo surgery before they mastered efficient voice production techniques. Protracted periods of aphonia can last several weeks to even months in these patients. Typically, return of useful conversational voice is expected within 4 weeks after surgery. Patients with emotional fear of voice can be helped with voice therapy. Patients are initiated on SOVT therapies and production techniques. For those with marked edema, this results in improvement over a 2–4-week period. For those with emotional fear of voice production, return to voice is usually quicker.

Durability of the Procedure

Patients should avoid elective intubation for at least 2 months following surgery since placement of an endotracheal tube risks disruption of the integrity of the healing neo-commissure. Once the neo-commissure has mucosalized and healed, subsequent intubations should ideally be performed with a 6.0 or smaller endotracheal tube with a grade I view to avoid any trauma to the anterior glottic web. Maintaining the integrity and sharp "V" of the neo-commissure is our best chance of creating symmetric vibratory patterns with complete closure. Such healing is compromised if the anterior glottic web is disrupted at any point postoperatively. After disruption, the neo-commissure can heal in a rounded fashion as opposed to in the ideal sharp "V." Rounding of the anterior commissure can result in closure disruption either from abnormal geometry or scar tissue formation. In such cases, the leak of air from failure of glottic closure and/or vibratory asymmetry results in increased breathiness, roughness, and loss of volume. If needed, the web can be revised with modest lengthening by repeating the same steps performed for the initial modified Wendler glottoplasty.

We aim to follow our patients for 1 year and have followed many for over 1 year after their surgeries. Pitch elevation remains stable, and voice satisfaction of self-reported voice outcomes appears to remain improved.

References

1. Casado JC, Rodriguez-Parra MJ, Adrian JA. Voice feminization in male-to-female transgendered clients after wendler's glottoplasty with vs. without voice therapy support. Eur Arch Otorhinolaryngol. 2017;274(4):2049–58. https://doi.org/10.1007/s00405-016-4420-8.
2. Kim HT. Vocal feminization for transgender women: current strategies and patient perspectives. Int J Gen Med. 2020;13:43–52. https://doi.org/10.2147/IJGM.S205102.
3. Schwarz K, Fontanari AMV, Schneider MA, et al. Laryngeal surgical treatment in transgender women: a systematic review and meta-analysis. Laryngoscope. 2017;127(11):2596–603. https://doi.org/10.1002/lary.26692.
4. Brown SK, Chang J, Hu S, et al. Addition of Wendler glottoplasty to voice therapy improves trans female voice outcomes. Laryngoscope. 2020; https://doi.org/10.1002/lary.29050.
5. Smith BE, Kempster GB, Sims HS. Patient factors related to voice therapy attendance and outcomes. J Voice. 2010;24(6):694–701. https://doi.org/10.1016/j.jvoice.2009.03.004.

Chapter 17
Feminization Laryngoplasty

James P. Thomas

Introduction

The guiding principle behind Feminization laryngoplasty is to convert the upper portions of the larynx to a more female morphology. The thyroid cartilage and pharynx are shortened vertically. The true and false vocal cords are shortened by removing the anterior portions. Below the glottis, the cricoid cartilage remains unchanged.

The target audience for feminization laryngoplasty is an individual whose comfortable speaking pitch is about 6–7 semitones too low for their preferred gender. Our approach for performing feminization laryngoplasty is to match our surgical intervention with each individual patient's goals. For some individuals, changing the voice is the primary transgender intervention that matters, even more so than physical appearance, as patients may have an obvious and very deep masculine voice that easily misgenders them. It is therefore critical that physicians and healthcare providers avoid assumptions about a patient's goals and instead inquire what the patient's specific goals are for their voice.

Some individuals have high vocal demands, perhaps singing for a career, and need to weigh the risk to their singing voice versus any benefit to their comfortable speaking pitch and loss of lower range. This concept is critical to stress to patients with high vocal demands as feminization laryngoplasty will result in the loss of vocal power and a reduction in overall vocal pitch range.

J. P. Thomas (✉)
Laryngology, Voicedoctor Private Practice, Portland, OR, USA
e-mail: thomas@voicedoctor.net

M. S. Courey et al. (eds.), *Voice and Communication in Transgender and Gender Diverse Individuals*, https://doi.org/10.1007/978-3-031-24632-6_17

Preoperative Assessment

Vocal Examination

We perform and record a vocal capabilities assessment on every patient. This assessment includes a battery of vocal tasks including comfortable speaking pitch, lowest pitch, highest pitch, maximum phonation time, high-volume task, low-volume singing task, and vegetative sounds such as cough or throat clear.

At a minimum, daily speaking pitch plays a role in sounding feminine, and this measure is often the voice that patients find most important. Since determining a comfortable speaking pitch especially at the time of a physical examination can prove elusive, our goal is to determine an approximate median note within a range of notes that an individual uses in casual conversation. Most individuals have some melody to their speaking voice and consequently use a range of several notes during typical and comfortable conversation. More emotional circumstances drive changes in pitch which can complicate the vocal assessment.

During our assessment, we record the patient reading a standard passage while assessing the voice for the middle note of their conversational voice. Usually patients will demonstrate a predominant pitch, but in cases where the latter is difficult to find, we assess the pitch at the end of their phrases. We will often ask individuals to speak in both their best feminine voice and in their "old, more classically cis-male" voice to elicit a range of comfortable speaking pitch tasks.

Consequently, there are times during an examination when casual, non-elicited conversation reveals a different comfortable speaking pitch. This casual voice may come closest to the true comfortable speaking pitch. Overall, comfortable speaking pitch is an imprecise yet useful measure.

An additional technique we incorporate into our vocal capabilities assessment is the use of musical notation from piano. It is incredibly important to assess the lowest note that an individual can reach both before and after an intervention. And while it can be very difficult to discriminate the cause of a change in the comfortable speaking pitch (surgery, training, mood), a change in the lowest note is almost certainly due to the intervention.

Role of Preoperative Therapy: Is it Indicated? Is there a Role?

Voice therapy can be thought of as a low-risk intervention, especially when compared to surgical intervention. It probably does no direct harm to the human voice. Individuals who attempt voice therapy and succeed to their satisfaction can be extremely happy. At the very least, voice therapy can be complementary to any surgery as there is no current surgery which alters the entire vocal tract to the point where it is structurally female. It is certainly reasonable to explain the role of voice therapy to all patients and to offer it to anyone seeking voice modifications.

Still, we cannot go so far as to say that voice therapy should be required for everyone considering feminization laryngoplasty. After successful surgery with feminization laryngoplasty, many individuals need no further intervention. Internally they already identify as female, and their vocal behaviors are already feminine so that after surgery they cannot access a male voice even with true effort.

Surgical Technique

1. Surgery is typically under general anesthesia, although it is possible under local anesthesia as well. General anesthesia avoids patient movement while sewing the true vocal cords back together. A 6.0 endotracheal tube is inserted with the cuff inferior to the cricoid cartilage. This avoids mucosal tearing and cuff rupture during removal of the anterior thyroid cartilage.
2. The surgical approach is external, incising the neck parallel to the relaxed skin tension lines typically over the upper thyroid cartilage. The platysma is raised superiorly and inferiorly exposing the anterior half of each thyroid ala (laterally to the insertion of the thyrohyoid muscle, superiorly to the hyoid bone, and inferiorly to the cricoid cartilage).
3. The upper wing of each thyroid cartilage is separated from the surrounding soft tissue attachments. Eight to ten millimeter, measured from the apex, is removed from the superior thyroid cartilage with a knife or saw depending upon calcification and overall size of the cartilage. The remaining thyroid cartilage should approximate a female cartilage height for the same height individual, so adjustments in this measurement are adaptable to overall body size. This increases the gap between the thyroid cartilage and hyoid bone and allows further elevation of the thyroid cartilage in the neck to shorten the pharynx.
4. Depending on the width and the angulation of the anterior thyroid cartilage, vertical cuts between 1 and 6 mm on either side of midline allow removal of the central thyroid cartilage. Remove more for larger thyroid cartilage and less for smaller thyroid cartilage. A typical amount would be to make cuts about 3 mm either side of midline which end up removing a central strut about 4 mm wide. The kerf of the cuts is about 1 mm for the saws I use.

   These cuts allow the thyroid cartilage to angle more medially, leading to smaller internal dimensions at the level of the glottis. They reduce the projection of the thyroid cartilage much more than any "tracheal shave," the cosmetic procedure to reduce the visual projection of the Adam's apple. The cuts should be angled to allow for airtight closure after vocal cord shortening. Typically the larynx has not been entered yet, or if it has, it is a small perforation at the anterior portion of the laryngeal ventricles.
5. Opening up into the laryngeal ventricle separates the false from the true vocal cords. Stretching the false vocal cords, approximately 5 mm of each anterior false cord is excised, narrowing the supraglottis.

6. Before dividing the anterior commissure, the vocal ligaments are grasped, and the true vocal cords stretched. A marking suture is placed around the vocal ligament on each side. Typically this is placed at the 50% portion of the members' vocal cord measured between the anterior commissure and the vocal process. These marking sutures both define the new anterior dimension of the membranous vocal cord and keep track of the vertical dimension of the true vocal cord by defining the medial margin (Figs. 17.1 and 17.2).

   Without a marking suture, a true vocal cord that is allowed to retract after division can be difficult to reconstruct precisely. The mucosa may contract posteriorly to the vocal ligament. The vocal ligament can be difficult to distinguish among other tissues. Without a marking suture, reconstruction is more likely to be anatomically incorrect in some dimension.
7. Approximately the anterior 40% of the true vocal cord, including the mucosa, the vocal ligament, and a portion of the thyroarytenoid muscle, are removed. If the thyroarytenoid muscle is quite bulky, additional muscle may be removed by tensioning the muscle.

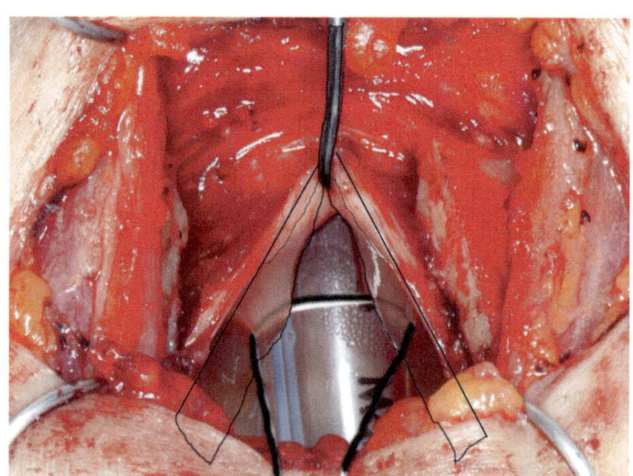

Fig. 17.1 View of true vocal cords after tension-marking suture is placed

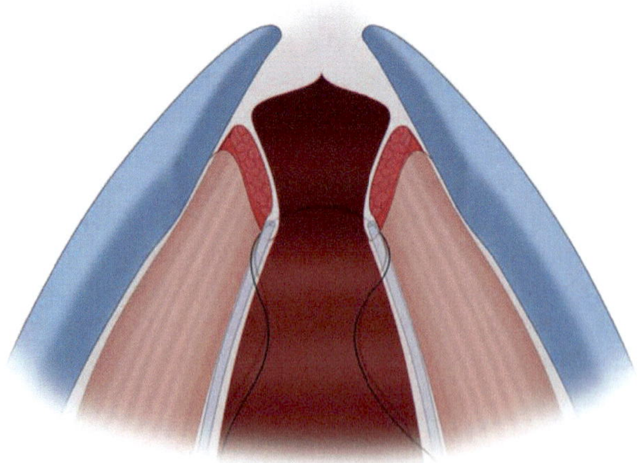

Fig. 17.2 View of marking suture still in place after excision of anterior true vocal cords

8. By placing tension on the marking suture to mimic the new anterior commissure and stretching the true vocal cords, the new anterior commissure should not extend past the inner thyroid lamina on either side. Otherwise the remaining true vocal cord will lack tension when the thyroid cartilage is re-approximated (Fig. 17.3a,b).
9. A series of approximately 1 mm holes are drilled in the hyoid bone and along the superior margins of the thyroid cartilage for elevation of the larynx. Two holes are placed along the medial cut edges of the thyroid cartilage for reconstruction of the anterior larynx.
10. All sutures are placed into position before any tightening is done. 0-Ethibond braided sutures are used to elevate the thyroid cartilage. A total of four sutures are placed through the thyroid ala and the hyoid bone for even elevation (Fig. 17.4).

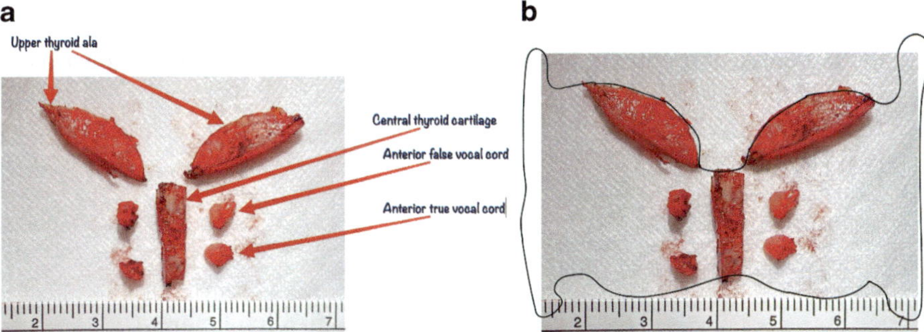

Fig. 17.3 (**a**, **b**) Removal of the cartilage and soft tissue

Fig. 17.4 Placement of drill holes

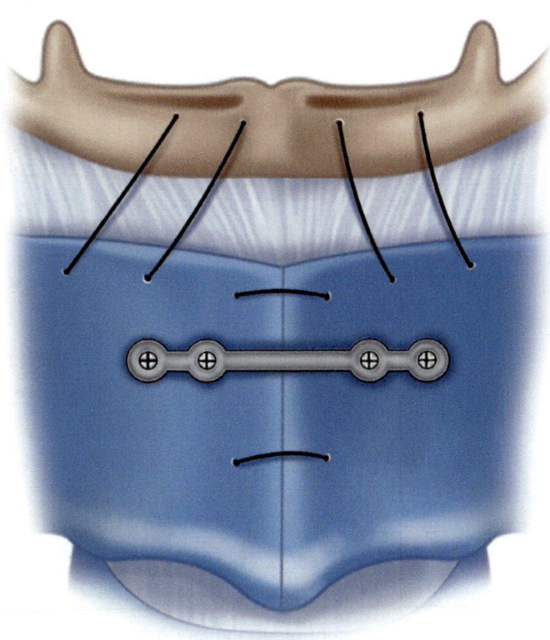

11. To reconstruct the glottis, Gore-Tex CV-5 suture creates a new anterior commissure. I use two opposing horizontal mattress sutures. The first suture enters the left thyroarytenoid muscle, vocal ligament, and vocal mucosa into the airway. It then enters the opposite right vocal cord through the mucosa, ligament, and a portion of thyroarytenoid muscle. The suture then returns on a similar path perhaps 1 mm inferior for a unilateral horizontal mattress suture that recreates an anterior commissure (Fig. 17.5). For balance and security, a second Gore-Tex suture is placed in apposition, starting with and exiting the right vocal cord.
12. A 4-0 Monocryl suture is passed through the central portion of the thyroarytenoid muscle to direct reattachment of the muscle to the cut edge and inner lamina of the thyroid cartilage. I loop the suture twice through the muscle for security. The suture is brought out along the cut edge of the thyroid cartilage, passed into a hole several millimeters from the edge of the cartilage and back out through another hole, and then tightened. This has the effect of reattaching the thyroarytenoid muscle to the most medial portion of the thyroid cartilage (Fig. 17.6a,b).

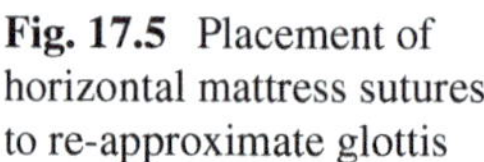

Fig. 17.5 Placement of horizontal mattress sutures to re-approximate glottis

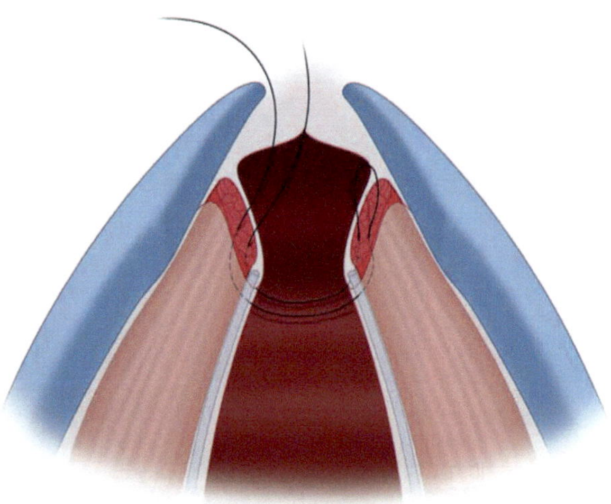

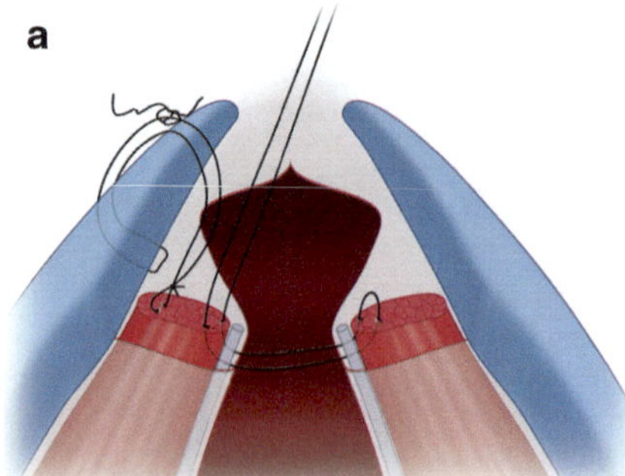

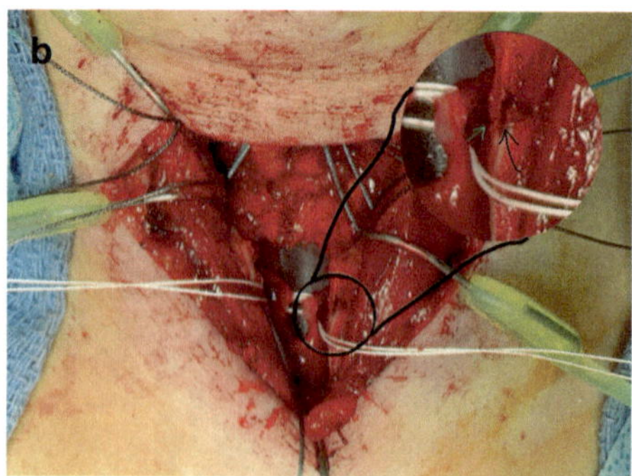

Fig. 17.6 (**a**, **b**) Placement of monofilament suture for tension of thyroarytenoid muscle

13. 13. For thyroid cartilage closure, an absorbable 4-0 monofilament (Monocryl) suture is placed through the upper holes in the superior thyroid cartilage and internally includes the cut edges of the false vocal cords with the intent of pulling the false cords against the upper, inner thyroid lamina during closure. This needle remains attached temporarily.
14. A similar 4-0 absorbable suture is passed through the inferior thyroid cartilage holes and includes the cut edge of the subglottic mucosa, again with the intent that the mucosa will reattach to the inner thyroid perichondrium and that there will be an airtight seal in the immediate postoperative period. The needle also remains attached temporarily.
15. As the thyroid cartilage is re-approximated, the Gore-Tex sutures are monitored, keeping them near the intended level for the new anterior commissure. The upper Monocryl suture is passed through the base of the epiglottis, pulling it tight against the upper thyroid cartilage cut edge for an airtight closure. Similarly, the lower Monocryl suture is passed through the cricothyroid membrane, snugging it up against the inferior thyroid cartilage, again for an airtight closure.
16. A four-hole, linear plate is bent to the shape of the newly angled anterior thyroid cartilage. It is placed preferably at the same level as the original attachment of the anterior commissure, typically about 10 mm superior to the inferior thyroid cartilage margin. Four-millimeter, self-tapping screws are placed bilaterally. The Gore-Tex sutures, which are slippery, can be pulled and snugged between the coapted edges of thyroid cartilage, tightened, and tied around the plate to maintain the new anterior commissure against the inner thyroid perichondrium. I have attempted to monitor this tightening internally with a flexible endoscope but have been unsuccessful in visualizing it while tightening it. Consequently, the tightening is based on feel, desiring tension, but not wanting to pull through and tear the mucosa through which the suture passes.
17. The Ethibond sutures are tightened, elevating the thyroid cartilage in the neck. There typically still remains a several millimeter gap between the thyroid cartilage and hyoid bone after tying the sutures.
18. The strap muscles are re-approximated in the midline with monofilament absorbable suture. One to three inverted sutures close the platysma layer and a running, subcuticular, monofilament absorbable suture, with no knots, re-approximates the epithelium. Cyanoacrylate glue seals the skin.

Postoperative Management

Recovery Room

Out of the 250 individuals on whom we have performed feminization laryngoplasty, two patients developed negative pressure pulmonary edema postoperatively in the recovery room. These patients were both successfully managed with diuretics and close observation.

Initial 3 Days

The most critical risk in the postoperative period is infection with concomitant excess supraglottic mucosal swelling and airway obstruction. All surgeries are performed as an outpatient at a surgery center. We then examine the patient in the clinic daily for 3 days with an endoscope.

Infection risk is managed by preoperative administration of clindamycin and a third-generation cephalosporin (or a fluoroquinolone in penicillin allergic patients). A cephalosporin or fluoroquinolone is continued orally for 7 days after surgery. In a typical postoperative course, there is mild post-arytenoid, supraglottic swelling on the first postoperative day. This increases to moderate post-arytenoid mucosal edema on the second postoperative day. This begins to diminish on the third postoperative day. In cases of infection, the swelling typically increases again on the third postoperative day.

None of our patients have demonstrated airway obstruction at the level of the glottis. Even very swollen true vocal cords do not significantly restrict the airway. A restricted airway can easily occur from post-arytenoid supraglottic swelling. The redundant mucosa is drawn over the arytenoid cartilages into the laryngeal introitus during inspiration.

Neck infection can be mitigated by decompressing any fluid accumulation that might represent infection externally with a drain. A Medrol dose pack or other steroids can be given. An impaired airway can be managed by a temporary tracheostomy in extreme cases. However, by instituting the current preoperative antibiotic regimen, postoperative antibiotics, and the serial 3-day monitoring, infections have tended to be non-urgent. Somewhat indolent infections have still appeared a few weeks later and required further antibiotic management and/or hardware/suture removal.

Subcutaneous emphysema from incomplete surgical sealing or high subglottic pressure can be treated with a drain. Observation works for very small amounts of crepitus.

Patients viewing their swollen vocal cords during the initial postoperative period are typically curious how their voice will turn out. We have not been able to correlate visual findings of edema or ecchymosis during this period with ultimate voice outcomes. Some individuals swell more than others. This initial postoperative monitoring is really only for early identification of postoperative infection. Diminished supraglottic edema on day 3 is the indication that patients may safely travel home.

Voice Use

We recommend 2 weeks of voice rest. Patients likely never completely comply with voice rest as they all perform some degree of throat clearing, coughing up of secretions or blood, talking in their sleep, or forgetting and making sounds. While we cannot prove that this sound production has not loosened a vocal cord, it does not seem common.

Expected Outcomes: Healing Phase, Return to Voice Production, and Durability of the Procedure

Healing Phase: Voice

At 2 weeks postoperative, some individuals can produce voice. More commonly, the vocal cords remain swollen or stiff and making the vocal cords vibrate gradually returns over the next few weeks. The initial voice is often rough and at a low pitch given the vocal cord swelling.

We ask patients not to strain or lift more than 10 pounds for 1 month after surgery. The only known probable vocal cord tear seemed to occur in an individual who was singing forcefully at 3 weeks after surgery, and her pitch suddenly dropped when she felt a pop.

We assess the voice at 2 months postoperatively by having the patient record a vocal capability assessment on their phone or computer, similar to the one obtained in the voice lab before surgery. The patient often reports that the pitch is gradually rising over the preceding weeks.

In cases where the voice remains impaired at 2 months, there's a strong possibility that a granuloma has formed near the anterior commissure and is pressing on the vocal cords, dampening vibrations. If there is an option to remove it in the office, manually or with a laser, voice restoration is quicker, and the risk that the granuloma will leave an anterior vocal cord gap is reduced.

After 2 months, the pitch continues to rise slightly, and some roughness may smooth out spontaneously. More severe roughness that is present 2–3 months after surgery can often be managed with an office KTP laser mucosal tightening procedure to correct asymmetry between the true vocal cords. Feedback from patients suggests that the voice seems to completely stabilize by about 9 months after surgery. These observations may be from a combination of ongoing tightening of the vocal cords during healing as well as the patient learning to use the new shorter vocal cord length.

Although the goal of Feminization laryngoplasty is to achieve a feminine voice after a single procedure, this does not preclude revision surgery for inadequate pitch elevation nor preclude laser tuneups of the voice for additional improvement or correction of a complication. There are various pathways to achieve the patient's goal of a natural feminine voice.

An office KTP laser has proven very useful for postoperative tuning. If there is a mild asymmetry between the two vocal cords, the individual may have roughness in their upper singing range. The KTP laser can tighten the superior surface of the vocal cord and straighten a slightly convex membranous vibratory vocal cord margin as it heals. A bilateral treatment of the superior surface vocal cord mucosa can at times increase the pitch by another semitone.

For asymmetries that are too large for the KTP laser, or for incomplete pitch elevation, a return to surgery using microlaryngeal CO_2 laser techniques can further de-bulk the now shortened true vocal cord. For individuals with a very thick vocal cord, this is a better approach than over-shortening the true vocal cord initially. An extremely short, but still massive/thick vocal cord will vibrate at a high pitch, but the individual will have almost limited volume.

One approach is to remove thyroarytenoid muscle mass. Another non-exclusive approach is to reduce the vertical height of the vibratory margin.

Both the office KTP laser and the surgical CO_2 laser treatments are also effective management in individuals who have had vocal cord webbing and may have inadequate pitch elevation or excessive air leak from convex membranous vocal cord margins.

Durability of the Procedure

Among our cohort of patients, we have 15 patients who have demonstrated 10–17 years of follow-up. Their voices appear to have remained stable after initial phases of healing. In two studies (Macmillan, Nuyen [accepted 2021]), more than 180 patients have been followed for a median of 16 months. While results in terms of pitch are on a bell curve with a median gain of 6 semitones at the comfortable speaking pitch and a median removal of 7 semitones from the low end of the vocal range, there is one case of deterioration of pitch over a year after surgery. We suspect that infection may have caused necrosis of the thyroid cartilage at the plate with subsequent loss of anterior commissure suspension of the true vocal cord.

Conclusions

Treatment of the voice, in an individual desiring an elevation of comfortable speaking pitch and vocal range, is a process that may include more than one intervention. Some combination of surgery and training for shortening the vocal cords, de-bulking of the thyroarytenoid muscle, tightening of the mucosa, elevation of the larynx, and narrowing the pharynx can lead to a natural female voice. In an ideal scenario, this could be a single procedure. In other individuals it may be only voice therapy. However, in some individuals, it may be a custom process depending on goals, surgical outcomes, and therapy responsiveness. It is possible for many individuals to achieve their vocal goal of matching their voice with their gender identity.

Further Reading

Nuyen BA, Qian ZJ, Campbell RD, Erickson-DiRenzo E, Thomas J, Sung CK. Feminization Laryngoplasty: 17-year review on long-term outcomes, safety, and technique. Otolaryngol Head Neck Surg. 2021;1945998211036870. https://doi.org/10.1177/01945998211036870. Epub ahead of print. PMID: 34399638.

Kunachak S, Prakunhungsit S, Sujjalak K. Thyroid cartilage and vocal fold reduction: a new phonosurgical method for male-to-female transsexuals. Ann Otol Rhinol Laryngol. 2000;109:1082–6.

Thomas JP, Macmillan C. Feminization laryngoplasty: assessment of surgical pitch elevation. Eur Arch Otorhinolaryngol. 2013;270(10):2695–700. https://doi.org/10.1007/s00405-013-2511-3. Epub 2013 Apr 30. PMID: 23632870.

Chapter 18
Type III Thyroplasty: Voice Masculinization

Vyas Prasad and Marc Remacle

Introduction

Isshiki described the type III thyroplasty for patients requiring pitch lowering not amenable or responsive to voice therapy. His indications for this intervention were for males with high vocal pitch, and 'a type of dysphonia characterized by a high pitch and a breathy voice (mutational falsetto). The laryngeal appearance in these patients includes a narrow posterior glottic gap and a small amplitude of vibration, suggesting a stiff vocal fold [1–4]. In recent years, the indications for type III thyroplasty, with minor variations on the original technique, have been extended to include transgender male patients who, despite androgen and voice therapy, are unable to achieve congruence between voice and physical appearance. The results for modified type III thyroplasty have been published [5]. These principles for this surgical intervention are in keeping with the physics and physiology for voice production and have been modified by various other laryngologists over time.

This chapter will present concepts for masculinization of voice; a background of therapy with a focus on the authors experience in therapies, pitfalls, and pearls from surgery; and a discussion on future improvements.

V. Prasad
Singapore Medical Specialist Centre, Otolaryngology-Head and Neck Surgery, Singapore, Singapore

M. Remacle (✉)
Department of ORL-Head & Neck Surgery, Centre Hospitalier Luxembourg—Eich, Luxembourg, Luxembourg

M. S. Courey et al. (eds.), *Voice and Communication in Transgender and Gender Diverse Individuals*, https://doi.org/10.1007/978-3-031-24632-6_18

Background

Hormone replacement therapy has historically been the primary treatment for transgender male patients. Androgen therapy alters the secondary sexual characteristics with alteration in hair pattern, fat and muscle distribution, and voice. The alteration to voice, due to thickening of the vocal fold mucosa and hypertrophy of the laryngeal musculature, is irreversible. In some transgender men, however, these changes are not sufficient to lower pitch satisfactorily. In addition, for personal and other health reasons, some transgender men are unable to receive androgen therapy. Often, these transgender male patients find themselves still being perceived as female when they speak despite all other attributes being masculine [6, 7]. Surgery for voice masculinization, therefore, is rare compared to feminization and is performed when the patient has a feminine voice due to an inability take androgen therapy or when the response to androgen therapy is suboptimal.

Preoperative Assessment

A thorough history and examination of the patient undergoing voice surgery is mandatory with input by an endocrinologist and psychologist where necessary. Prior videolaryngostroboscopic (VLS) examination of the patient with recording facilities for comprehensive documentation is very useful. Voice assessment is evaluated and while several protocols—local, national or international exist, we utilize the European Laryngological Society's Committee on Phoniatrics [8]. This is a multidimensional set of minimal basic measurements suitable for 'common' dysphonias. It consists of five different categories: perception (grade, roughness, breathiness), videostroboscopy (closure, regularity, mucosal wave and symmetry), acoustics (jitter, shimmer, F0-range and softest intensity), aerodynamics (phonation quotient) and subjective rating (Voice Handicap Index, VHI; Visual Analogue Scale, VAS).

The lowering of pitch when pressure is applied to the anterior thyroid cartilage backwards during phonation (manual or Gutzmann pressure test) should lower the pitch and may predict success from relaxation thyroplasty [4].

Voice Questionnaires

Several voice questionnaires have been used in transgender patients including gender nonspecific ones such as the Voice Handicap Index and Voice-Related Quality of Life (VR-QOL) [9, 10]. The Transgender Self-Evaluation Questionnaire (TSEQ) was the progenitor of transgender self-administered questionnaires adapted from the well-established VHI. Thereafter, the Transsexual Voice Questionnaire (TVQ^{MtF}) was developed from the TSEQ and is a validated patient-reported outcome measurement tool consisting of three categories: anxiety and avoidance, gender identity and voice quality. A lower total score reflects a better outcome [11, 12]. The TVQ^{MtF} is a MtF questionnaire however. There is a significant paucity in the literature of FtM questionnaire-based studies despite the fact that androgen therapy is not always successful and this group of patients do indeed benefit of voice therapy and surgery when indicated. It is postulated that the VHI and VR-QOL are used in this group.

Informed Consent

The management of patients is multidisciplinary, and all available options (medical, surgical and behavioural) should be explored and where possible offered. Some MtF patients respond well to voice and behavioural therapy and can function albeit with some difficulty in falsetto. Similarly, psychotherapy at a younger age has been shown to reduce the need for surgery in puberphonia. Botox injections have been explored to paralyse the cricothyroid muscle and lower the pitch as has injection laryngoplasty [13–15]. The aims of surgery and risks versus benefits are clearly explained, and it is worthwhile in selected cases for the patient to meet previously treated subjects.

Preoperative Voice Therapy: Is There a Role?

Voice therapy is an essential part of the management of patients who have committed to fully alter their gender. It aims to not only instruct the patient on how to manage their altered voices in various conversational settings but to master vocal cues, control of breathing, flow phonation, masculine cues, vocabulary and emotional aspects that are so intrinsically linked to perceptions of gender through voice [16]. In addition to the previously mentioned gender cues, vocal pitch may also be targeted in therapy. The fundamental frequency range for gender is well established. Culture, language, size of the individual (directly proportional to size of the vocal tract and inversely related to fundamental frequency) and account for the variation in fundamental frequency. There is also a range where fundamental frequency is shared between males and females, i.e. 145–165 Hz [10]. The ‘telephone test’ is often cited as a useful measure in assessing if the transgender patient has the vocal characteristics ascribed to the particular gender. It is a non-visual test and has been used to assess the success of therapeutic interventions [17].

Surgical Technique: Type III (Relaxation) Thyroplasty

This procedure is essentially a modified Isshiki type III (i.e. *IIIB anterior/paramedian relaxation thyroplasty* based on the European Laryngology Society classification system) [1–4, 18] (Fig. 18.1). Isshiki stated that the procedure should be performed strictly under local anaesthesia or under total intravenous anaesthesia with the patient spontaneously breathing and capable of being awakened to phonate, allowing for adjustment of the tension of the vocal folds. We prefer to perform the procedure under general anaesthesia using a laryngeal mask airway to allow for inspection of the larynx intra-operatively with a distal chip flexible nasendoscope with video recording capability.

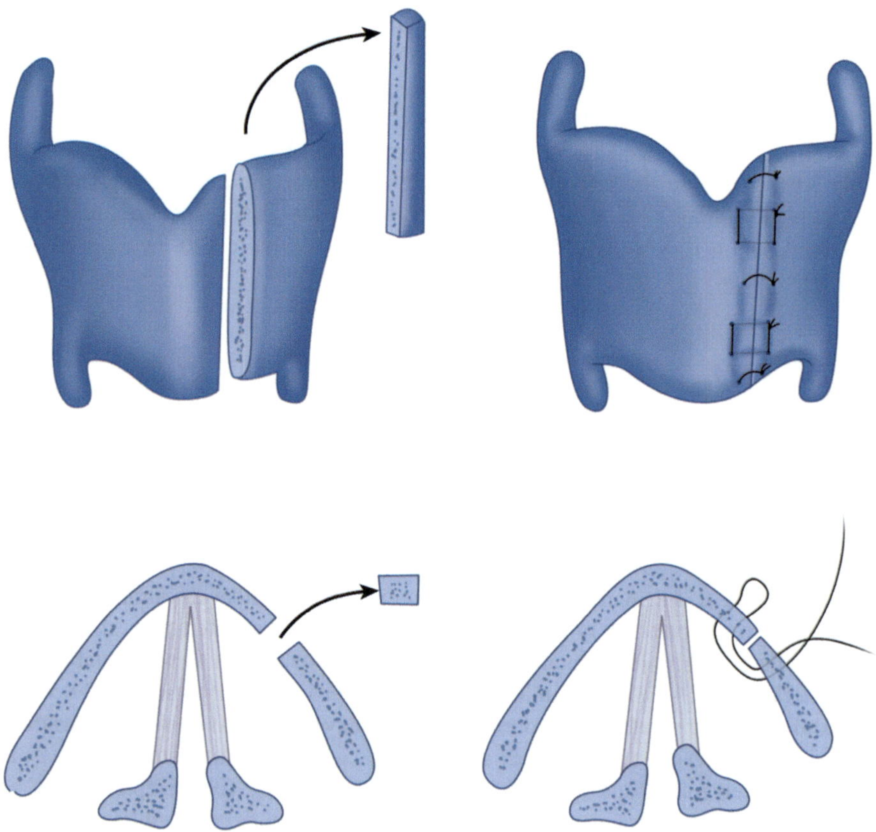

Fig. 18.1 Isshiki's thyroplasty type 3

The salient steps of this procedure as with most anterior neck procedures are as follows:

Step 1: Incise the skin in a horizontal neck crease where possible equidistant of the midline and at the lower border of the thyroid cartilage over the cricothyroid membrane.

Step 2: Skin flaps are raised, and the larynx is exposed up to the superior margin of the thyroid cartilage without the need to cut the strap muscles but merely separating them.

Step 3: The thyroid cartilage is cut vertically, 5 mm either side of the midline along the entire length. Important landmarks are the thyroid notch and the inferior rim of the thyroid cartilage. Calcified cartilage may require a fine side-end burr or a sagittal saw. The cuts extend through the outer perichondrium but do not transgress the inner perichondrium.

Step 4: The anterior 1 cm of inner perichondrium is carefully elevated from the posterior cartilage segment with the attached Broyles' ligament. This is retrodisplaced into the larynx, and the posterior segments are allowed to override it on either side laterally.

Step 5: Endoscopic evaluation of the larynx using the video endoscope is performed through the laryngeal mask (LMA). The degree of retrusion is noted.

Step 6: The segments of thyroid cartilage lateral to the anterior segment are secured in position over the middle segment with a non-absorbable mono-filament suture (Nylon 3–0).

Step 7: A small suction drain is inserted, and fibrin glue applied over the area of retrusion. This may be helpful in reducing any bleeding/haematoma formation (Figs. 18.2, 18.3, 18.4, 18.5, 18.6, 18.7).

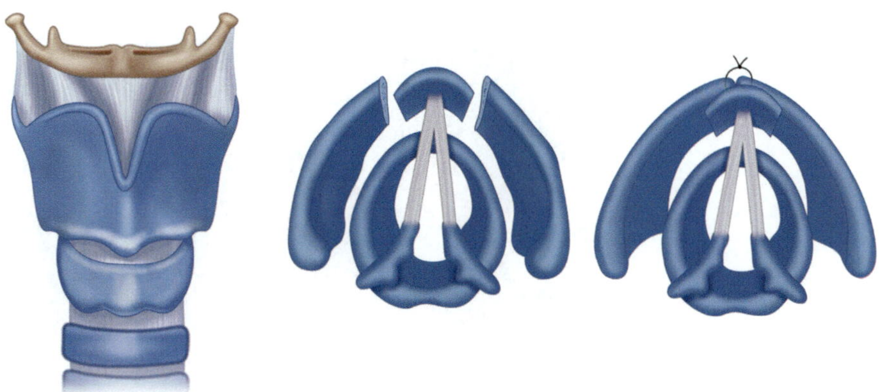

Fig. 18.2 Schematic diagram of relaxation thyroplasty type IIIB

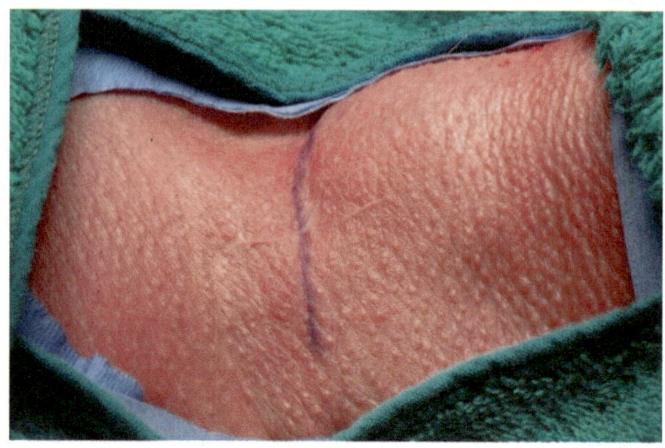

Fig. 18.3 Neck prepared with skin marking

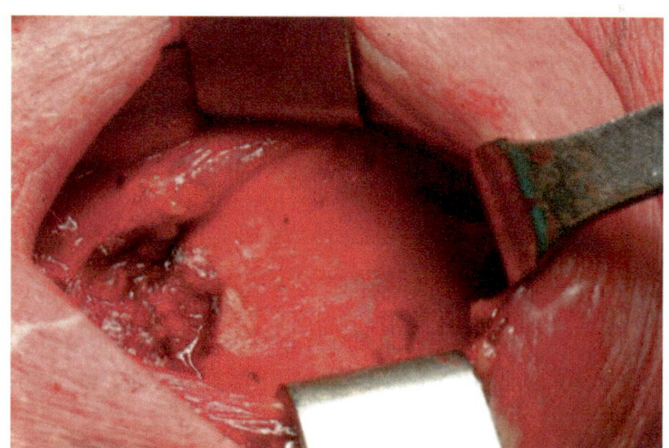

Fig. 18.4 Exposure of thyroid cartilage

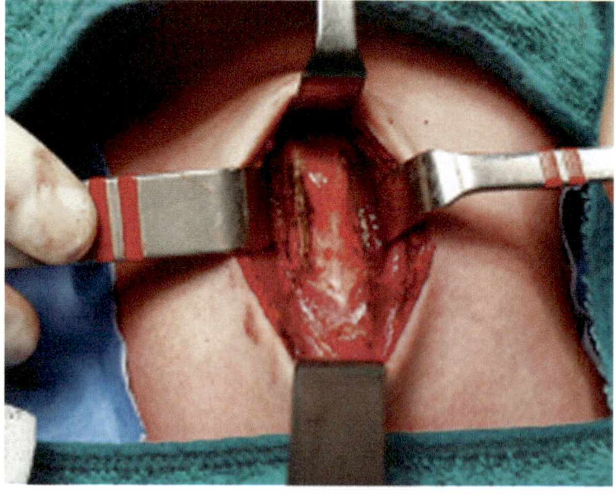

Fig. 18.5 Vertical incisions either side of midline

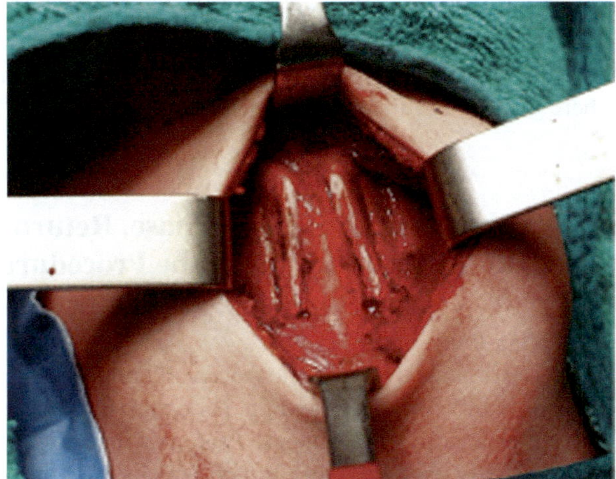

Fig. 18.6 Separation of anterior segment and elevation of inner perichondrium

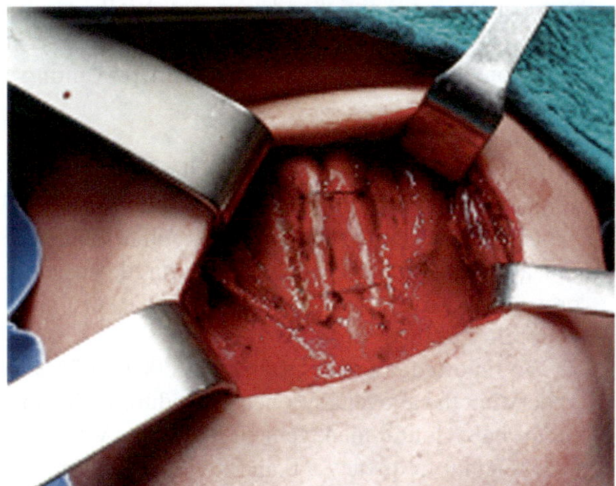

Fig. 18.7 Segments of thyroid cartilage secured in position

Postoperative Management

Patients are advised a week of low-intensity voicing after discharge and placed on a 5-day course of oral broad-spectrum antibiotics, steroid inhalers and proton-pump inhibitors empirically. Thereafter, patients undergo voice therapy after surgery to optimize the functional results with the new glottic configuration.

Patients who undergo any treatment for transgender voice are usually followed up in the multidisciplinary setting. Our experience is that most patients are better at gauging the success of their respective therapies, and in that regard, subjective questionnaires prove to be better yardsticks of therapeutic benefit as opposed to other non-patient-based assessments including acoustic and aerodynamic studies. The mere focus on their pitch range and fundamental frequency without taking into consideration formant frequencies, breathiness, prosody and their own overall subjective rating and satisfaction has been shown in several studies to be a poor yardstick for success. However, tests such as the 'telephone test' do have their place where gender identification is made on non-visual cues [8].

Expected Outcome: Healing Phase, Return to Voice Production and Durability of the Procedure

1. Healing Phase

   The drain is usually removed several hours after the procedure assuming that there is little drainage, and the surgical wound is left to heal accordingly with appropriate dressing changes. There may be a degree of vocal fold oedema, and this usually settles within a month. Fractures of the thyroid cartilage and haematomas have been described anecdotally. The vertical incisions if made to deep can tear the inner perichondrium, potentially resulting in hematoma and granuloma formation. Some authors advocate placing a silastic block to maintain the retrusion of the anterior segment and preventing the retruded segment from 'popping out' [19].
2. Return to Voice Production

   Patients undergo regular voice therapy sessions a week to a fortnight after surgery. They may have some issues with pitch breaks and instability which are generally amenable to voice therapy. Other aspects related to appropriate masculinization of their voices are also nurtured. These include vocal cues, breathing, prosody and so on. This process may take several months.
3. Durability of the Procedure

   We reported a small series from 2001 to 2008 on seven male patients who underwent the abovementioned procedure with a mean age of 21 years after failure of behavioural management. Outcome was assessed based on the change to fundamental frequency, F0 and the VHI. The mean fundamental frequency was lowered from 187 Hz to 104 Hz ($p < 0.001$), while the mean VHI improved from 70 to 21 [5]. We followed up our patients over an average of 17 months. Some patients continued to have vocal roughness for several weeks but with targeted voice therapy improved completely. Jitter and shimmer remained within the normal range.

References

1. Isshiki N, Morita H, Okamura H, Hiramoto M. Thyroplasty as a new phonosurgical technique. Acta Otolaryngol. 1974;78(5–6):451–7. https://doi.org/10.3109/00016487409126379.
2. Isshiki N, Taira T, Tanabe M. Surgical alteration of the vocal pitch. J Otolaryngol. 1983;12(5):335–40.

3. Isshiki N, Tanabe M, Ohkawa M, Kita M. Laryngeal framework surgery for voice disorders. Auris Nasus Larynx. 1985;12(Suppl 2):S217–20. https://doi.org/10.1016/s0385-8146(85)80062-6.
4. Isshiki N. Phonosurgery—theory and practice. Tokyo: Springer; 1989.
5. Remacle M, Matar N, Verduyckt I, Lawson G. Relaxation thyroplasty for mutational falsetto treatment. Ann Otol Rhinol Laryngol. 2010;119(2):105–9. https://doi.org/10.1177/000348941011900207.
6. Pan S, Honig SC. Gender-affirming surgery: current concepts. Curr Urol Rep. 2018;19(8):62. https://doi.org/10.1007/s11934-018-0809-9.
7. Defreyne J, T'Sjoen G. Transmasculine hormone therapy. Endocrinol Metab Clin N Am. 2019;48(2):357–75. https://doi.org/10.1016/j.ecl.2019.01.004.
8. DeJonckere PH, Crevier-Buchman L, Marie JP, Moerman M, Remacle M, Woisard V, European Research Group on the Larynx. Implementation of the European Laryngological Society (ELS) basic protocol for assessing voice treatment effect. Rev Laryngol Otol Rhinol (Bord). 2003;124(5):279–83.
9. Jacobson BH, Johnson A, Grywalsky C, et al. The voice handicap index (VHI): development and validation. Am J Speech Lang Pathol. 1997;6:66–70.
10. Hogikyan ND, Sethuraman G. Validation of an instrument to measure voice-related quality of life (VR-QOL). J Voice. 1999;13(4):557–69. https://doi.org/10.1016/s0892-1997(99)80010-1.
11. Dacakis G, Davies S, Oates JM, Douglas JM, Johnston JR. Development and preliminary evaluation of the transsexual voice questionnaire for male-to-female transsexuals. J Voice. 2013;27(3):312–20. https://doi.org/10.1016/j.jvoice.2012.11.005.
12. Dacakis G, Oates JM, Douglas JM. Further evidence of the construct validity of the transsexual voice questionnaire (TVQ^{MtF}) using principal components analysis. J Voice. 2017;31(2):142–8. https://doi.org/10.1016/j.jvoice.2016.07.001.
13. Pau H, Murty GE. First case of surgically corrected puberphonia. J Laryngol Otol. 2001;115(1):60–1. https://doi.org/10.1258/0022215011906821.
14. van den Broek EM, Vokes DE, Dorman EB. Bilateral in-office injection laryngoplasty as an adjunctive treatment for recalcitrant Puberphonia: a case report and review of the literature. J Voice. 2016;30(2):221–3. https://doi.org/10.1016/j.jvoice.2015.03.019.
15. Hamdan AL, Khalifee E, Ghanem A, Jaffal H. Injection laryngoplasty in patients with Puberphonia. J Voice. 2019;33(4):564–6. https://doi.org/10.1016/j.jvoice.2018.02.017.
16. Hancock AB, Garabedian LM. Transgender voice and communication treatment: a retrospective chart review of 25 cases. Int J Lang Commun Disord. 2013;48(1):54–65. https://doi.org/10.1111/j.1460-6984.2012.00185.
17. Meister J, Kühn H, Shehata-Dieler W, Hagen R, Kleinsasser N. Perceptual analysis of the male-to-female transgender voice after glottoplasty-the telephone test. Laryngoscope. 2017;127(4):875–81. https://doi.org/10.1002/lary.26110.
18. Friedrich G, de Jong FI, Mahieu HF, Benninger MS, Isshiki N. Laryngeal framework surgery: a proposal for classification and nomenclature by the Phonosurgery Committee of the European Laryngological Society. Eur Arch Otorhinolaryngol. 2001;258(8):389–96. https://doi.org/10.1007/s004050100375.
19. Slavit DH, Maragos NE, Lipton RJ. Physiologic assessment of Isshiki type III thyroplasty. Laryngoscope. 1990;100(8):844–8. https://doi.org/10.1288/00005537-199008000-00009.

Chapter 19
Thyroid Cartilage Reduction

Joseph Chang

Introduction

Thyroid cartilage reduction is an adjunctive surgery that is often considered in the course of transgender female voice care, although it is not intended to alter voice. Thyroid cartilage reduction, also known as thyroid chondroplasty, laryngochondroplasty, or more colloquially as the "trach shave," reduces the projection of the thyroid notch or Adam's apple, as a prominent thyroid notch is often considered a masculine feature. Reduction of the thyroid notch is performed by removing the anterosuperior aspect of the thyroid cartilage and can often be performed in conjunction with voice surgery.

The first descriptions of thyroid cartilage reduction in the transgender population date as far back as 1975 [1]. The procedure was initially devised to provide cosmetic reduction of the Adam's apple, or thyroid cartilage prominence, as patients had found that hormonal medical therapy used by transgender women to address secondary male sexual characteristics did not physically alter laryngeal framework. Subsequently, there have been a number of slight modifications to the technique including the use of drills to smooth the contour of the incised cartilage in 1989 [2] and use of intraoperative endoscopic guidance to identify surgical landmarks in 2008 [3].

Preoperative Assessment

Occasionally, patients presenting for transgender female voice care are noted to maintain a chin-tucked position. This is oftentimes a behavior adopted by the patient

J. Chang (✉)
Department of Otolaryngology- Head and Neck Surgery, University of Washington, Seattle, WA, USA
e-mail: jbchang@uw.edu

M. S. Courey et al. (eds.), *Voice and Communication in Transgender and Gender Diverse Individuals*, https://doi.org/10.1007/978-3-031-24632-6_19

to hide their thyroid cartilage prominence and may be an indication that the patient may benefit from thyroid cartilage reduction. Not surprisingly, the thyroid notch is most prominent in patients with thin necks. Those with sufficient submental soft tissue to obscure the thyroid notch may not notice a drastic change in neck appearance.

As with all neck surgeries, patients should be assessed for factors that may affect their wound healing including diabetes, smoking, medical conditions contributing to immunocompromise, and history of keloid formation. Particularly important is a history of prior surgery or trauma that may have altered the laryngeal cartilage. Thyroid cartilage reduction must be carefully considered in those with altered laryngeal anatomy as the surgery removes portions of the cartilaginous support of the larynx.

Finally, patients should be carefully counseled regarding the expected surgical outcomes. Surgery may not be appropriate in those with unrealistic expectations. The degree of cartilage that can be safely removed is limited by the location where the vocal folds attach to the thyroid cartilage (Fig. 19.1). Especially in patients with

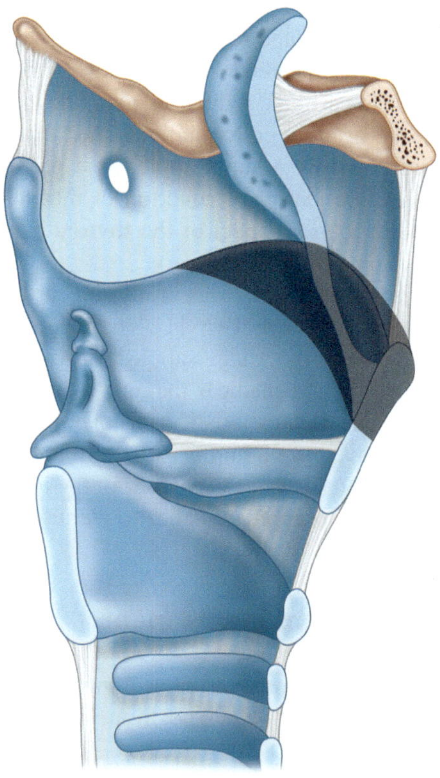

Fig. 19.1 Thyroid cartilage reduction. The anterosuperior aspect of the thyroid cartilage, shaded in gray, is removed to reduce the prominence of the thyroid notch. The degree of cartilage that can be removed is limited inferiorly by the location of the anterior vocal fold attachment. The residual thyroid alae should be shaped to mirror the shape of the natural thyroid cartilage contour

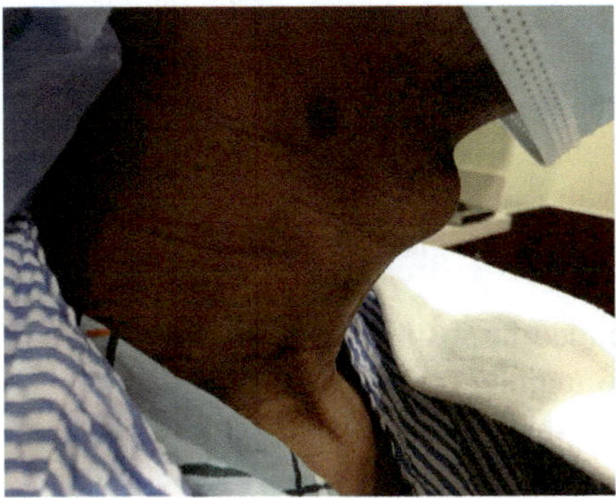
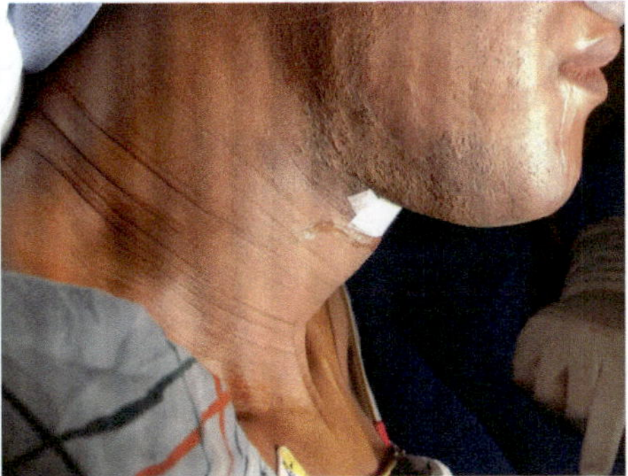

Fig. 19.2 Pre- and postoperative neck profile. The thyroid notch prominence may not be completely removed due to anatomical limitations. Paradoxically, the cricoid cartilage may become more visually noticeable after thyroid cartilage reduction. Postoperative edema may temporarily obscure the profile of the new thyroid notch after surgery. With resolution of the edema, the new thyroid prominence will become slightly more noticeable

thin necks, the thyroid prominence cannot be completely removed due to this anatomic limitation. Alternatively, in patients where sufficient thyroid cartilage can be removed, the prominence from the cricoid cartilage may become more dominant and noticeable (Fig. 19.2). Removal or reduction of the cricoid cartilage is not routinely performed.

Role of Preoperative Therapy

No preoperative voice therapy is necessary in isolated thyroid cartilage reduction surgery, as thyroid cartilage reduction is not intended to change the voice. A primary goal of the surgery is to leave enough thyroid cartilage in place that there are no changes to vocal fold mechanics including vocal fold tone, position, and movement. Large case series have confirmed the lack of postoperative dysphonia [3, 4].

Surgical Technique

Thyroid cartilage reduction is typically performed under general anesthesia especially when it is performed in conjunction with voice surgery. However, it can be completed under sedation and local anesthesia.

1. In the preoperative bay while the patient is sitting upright, a 3-cm cervical neck incision is marked out in a superior cervical skin crease that sits above the level of the thyroid notch. Ideally, the patient's cervicomental crease is used to help disguise the incision.

2. A laryngeal mask airway (LMA) is placed for ventilation by anesthesia, and the patient is placed in slight neck extension.
3. A flexible laryngoscope can be placed through the LMA and suspended above the patient's head to allow for direct visualization of the larynx on an external monitor throughout the case. Alternatively, the flexible laryngoscope can be placed by an assistant for a temporary view of the glottis when it comes time to identify the level of the vocal folds.
4. If a flexible laryngoscope is to be suspended in position throughout the case, a drape is placed over the laryngoscope to maintain the sterility of the field. The laryngoscope should be positioned such that the angulation control lever is accessible under the drape to allow the surgeon to adjust the view intraoperatively without violating sterile technique (Fig. 19.3).
5. The skin is incised, and subplatysmal dissection is carried inferiorly to the inferior border of the thyroid cartilage. The strap muscles are then divided in the midline to expose the thyroid cartilage.

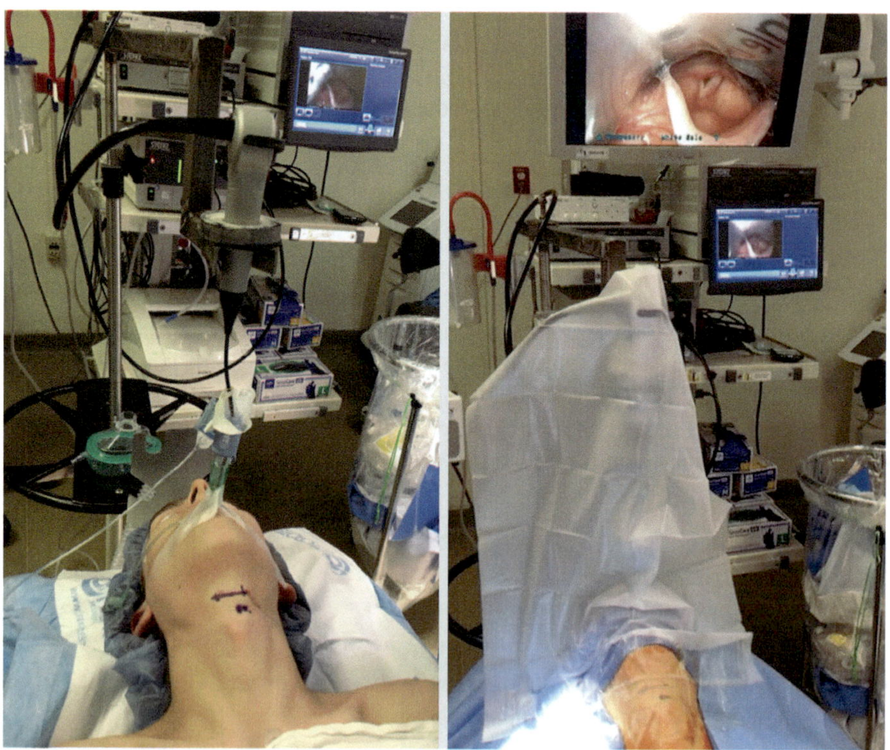

Fig. 19.3 Operating room configuration. A flexible laryngoscope is suspended above the patient with a view of the vocal folds and anterior laryngeal vestibule through a laryngeal mask airway. The patient is prepared and draped with the laryngoscope in place and oriented such that the angulation control lever of the laryngoscope is accessible to the surgeon through the drapes

6. A T-shaped incision is made in the thyroid perichondrium down the midline of the thyroid cartilage and along the superior margins of the thyroid alae. The perichondrium is then dissected off of the thyroid cartilage. A hook may be inserted in the thyroid notch to stabilize the larynx during the perichondrial dissection.
7. A needle is then placed in the midline of the thyroid cartilage into the laryngeal lumen to localize the attachment of the anterior commissure using the flexible laryngoscope for visual confirmation. This point is the lowest level at which thyroid cartilage can be removed.
8. The anterosuperior portions of the thyroid alae are then removed with a scalpel or drill, depending on the ossification of the cartilage, taking care to recreate the natural curvature of the superior border of the thyroid cartilage. It is important to bevel and smooth out the cartilage edges after alar resection.
9. The straps are then reapproximated in the midline to prevent postoperative tethering of the larynx to the skin, and then skin is closed.

The most critical step in this procedure is confirmation of the level of the vocal folds in step 7, as the consequences of over-excision and violation of the anterior commissure are severe. Even if the vocal folds are not directly injured, detachment of the vocal fold attachment to the thyroid cartilage can result in postoperative dysphonia and lowering of vocal pitch. Classically, the location of the anterior commissure is described as halfway between the thyroid notch and the inferior border of the thyroid cartilage. This anatomic guideline has been found to be unreliable with variation in anterior commissure location up to 4 mm above and 0.5 mm below this level [5, 6]. In a cadaveric study of 83 fresh larynges, 95% of men and 100% of women were found to have anterior commissures above the mid-thyroid cartilage line [5]. The use of this landmark will therefore frequently lure surgeons into over-excision of the cartilage. Given the desire to maximally reduce the thyroid prominence as well as to keep patients safe, it is prudent to confirm the location of the vocal fold with needle localization and laryngoscopic visualization in every patient.

Additional risks include injury to the superior laryngeal nerve with associated loss of laryngeal sensation and possible aspiration if dissection is carried too far laterally, as well as possible laryngeal fracture in the case of over aggressive cartilage removal. Fracture of the remaining inferior thyroid cartilage strut may result in vocal fold-level mismatch, vocal fold scarring, and loss of vocal fold tension with subsequent dysphonia and possible lowering of vocal pitch.

Postoperative Management

Postoperative management focuses primarily on incision care and prevention of scar formation. Patients should avoid any activities that put tension on the submental incision for at least 2 weeks. Depending on the method of incision closure, the incision may be exposed and can be cleaned regularly with saline or water and covered with ointment, such as Vaseline or Aquaphor. After 2 weeks, silicone gel or sheeting may be used on the scar to reduce scar hypertrophy and hyperpigmentation [7, 8].

Expected Outcomes

Beyond management of the incision and reduction of postoperative scarring, it is important to counsel patients regarding aesthetic outcomes and expectations in the healing phase. In the first few months after surgery, subcutaneous edema will help obscure the altered thyroid notch. As the edema resolves, the thyroid notch will become more visible.

As the voice should not be altered by isolated thyroid cartilage reduction, patients may return to full voice use after surgery with the caveat that some mild vocal fold swelling may occur due to inflammation from the adjacent surgery. If there is throat discomfort or worsening of the voice with prolonged talking, the patient should rest the voice until the discomfort and dysphonia resolve.

Quality of life has been shown to improve in transgender women after thyroid cartilage reduction (Tang 2020). However, this result reflects just one time point after surgery. There are currently no studies documenting long-term outcomes after thyroid cartilage reduction.

Conclusion

Although thyroid cartilage reduction is not intended to alter voice, it is often performed in conjunction with pitch elevation phonosurgery and is a helpful adjunct to improve quality of life in transgender women. While performing this surgery, it is important to localize the anterior commissure to maximize the degree to which the thyroid prominence can be reduced and to avoid detachment of the vocal folds with resultant dysphonia.

References

1. Wolfort FG, Parry RG. Laryngeal chondroplasty for appearance. Plast Reconstr Surg. 1975;56(4):371–4.
2. Wolfort FG, Dejerine ES, Ramos DJ, Parry RG. Chondrolaryngoplasty for appearance. Plast Reconstr Surg. 1990;86(3):464–9.
3. Spiegel JH, Rodriguez G. Chondrolaryngoplasty under general anesthesia using a flexible fiberoptic laryngoscope and laryngeal mask airway. Arch Otolaryngol Head Neck Surg. 2008;134(7):704–8. https://doi.org/10.1001/archotol.134.7.704.

4. Tang C. Evaluating patient benefit from laryngochondroplasty. Laryngoscope. 2020;130(Suppl 5):S1–S14. https://doi.org/10.1002/lary.29075.
5. Cinar U, Yigit O, Vural C, Alkan S, Kayaoglu S, Dadas B. Level of vocal folds as projected on the exterior thyroid cartilage. Laryngoscope. 2003;113(10):1813–6. https://doi.org/10.1097/00005537-200310000-00028.
6. Meiteles LZ, Lin PT, Wenk EJ. An anatomic study of the external laryngeal framework with surgical implications. Otolaryngol Head Neck Surg. 1992;106(3):235–40. https://doi.org/10.1177/019459989210600305.
7. Chan KY, Lau CL, Adeeb SM, Somasundaram S, Nasir-Zahari M. A randomized, placebo-controlled, double-blind, prospective clinical trial of silicone gel in prevention of hypertrophic scar development in median sternotomy wound. Plast Reconstr Surg. 2005;116(4):1013–20. https://doi.org/10.1097/01.prs.0000178397.05852.ce.
8. Cruz-Korchin NI. Effectiveness of silicone sheets in the prevention of hypertrophic breast scars. Ann Plast Surg. 1996;37(4):345–8. https://doi.org/10.1097/00000637-199610000-00001.

Index

A
Acceptance and Commitment Coaching (ACC), 127
Androgen supplementation, 13
Androgen therapy, 135
Anterior (Wendler) glottoplasty, 169
Anti-androgen supplementation, 11
Anti-androgen therapy, 9
Anti-transgender bias, 33
Antoni methods, 93–95
Anxiety and mental health management, 127, 128
Assigned female at birth (AFAB), 114, 115, 135
Assigned male at birth (AMAB), 114, 119

B
Biofeedback, 82
Breast cancer, 15
Breathy phonation, 66

C
Carbon dioxide laser, 172
Cepstral peak prominence (CPP), 50
Cepstral-spectral index of dysphonia (CSID), 50
Chest resonance, 82
Circumlaryngeal massage, 144
Cis-assumed, 29
Cisfemales, 80
Cisgender, 29
Cismales, 80
Clinician-perceived dysphonia, 46–47
CO_2 laser, 191, 205
Cognitive-behavioral therapy (CBT), 127
Consensus Auditory-Perceptual Evaluation of Voice (CAPE-V), 50, 163
Conversation training therapy (CTT), 73, 74
Cricothyroid approximation (CTA), 158, 161, 178
  expected outcomes, 167
  postoperative management, 166
  preoperative assessment, 162, 163
  preoperative therapy, 163, 164
  surgical technique, 164, 165
Cricothyroid, 116
CT-dominant, 116

D
Deadnaming, 38
Decision-making capacity, 23
Digital kymography, 180
Documented consent, 35

E
Embouchure, 116
Emotional tone of voice range, 96
Estradiol, 11
Estrogen-based HRT, 126, 127
Estrogen-based therapy, 9
Estrogen supplementation, 11
Ethinyl estradiol, 11
Evidence-based practice (EBP), 43
Excess pressure, 117
Exogenous androgen therapy, 135
Expressed consent, 35

M. S. Courey et al. (eds.), *Voice and Communication in Transgender and Gender Diverse Individuals*, https://doi.org/10.1007/978-3-031-24632-6

External androgen therapy, 136
Eye gaze, 106

F
Facial expression, 105
Female to male (FTM), 12–14
Feminization laryngoplasty, 158, 197
  outcomes, 205, 206
  postoperative management, 203, 204
  preoperative assessment, vocal examination, 198
  preoperative therapy, 198, 199
  surgical techniques, 199–203
Feminizing hormone therapy, 14, 21
Fertility preservation, 8, 9
Flipped voice, 116
Flow phonation (FP), 66, 69
  from structured tasks to generalization, 72
  pitfalls, 74
  practice and maintenance, 75, 76
Flow resistance tubes (FRT), 67
Forward resonance, 82
  hierarchy of tasks for, 83, 84
  techniques to, 81
4-point Likert scale, 48
Fundamental frequency (F0), 138, 139

G
Gender affirming voice care, 74
Gender-affirming voice surgery, 52, 53
Gender affirming voice therapy, 21, 75
Gender-affirming voice work, 44
Gender dysphoria, 8, 9, 20
  in adults and adolescents, 20
  behavioral and surgical treatment for, 17, 18
  definition of, 17
Gender expression, 142
Genderfluid person, 29
Gender identity, 8, 29, 31
Genderqueer person, 29
Glottal attacks, 116
Glottoplasty, 17–19, 22
Grade, roughness, breathiness, asthenia and strain (GRBAS) score, 50, 163

H
Habilitative vocal training, 117
Haptics, 106
Hard glottal attack, 116
Healing phase, 173, 195, 205, 206, 214
High-speed laryngoscopy, 180
Hormone replacement therapy, 208
Hormone therapy, 8, 9, 21
  for transgender individuals, 9
  for transgender men, 13, 14
  for transgender women, 9–12
Hybrid voice, 122

I
I, 127
Implied consent, 35
Informed consent, 36, 209
Internalized transphobia, 33
Intonation, 94, 140, 146, 147
Isshiki's thyroplasty type 3, 210

K
Kinetics, 106

L
Language, 141, 142, 146, 147
Laryngeal mask airway (LMA), 220
Laryngeal Reposturing with Voicing, 144
Laryngochondroplasty, *see* Thyroid cartilage reduction
Laryngoscopy, 114
Laryngostroboscopy, 173
Laser ablation, 181
Laser-assisted voice adjustment (LAVA), 169, 170
  outcomes
    durability of procedure, 174
    healing phase, 173
    return to voice production, 173, 174
  postoperative management, 173
  preoperative assessment, 170
  preoperative voice therapy, 171
  surgical techniques, 171–173
Laser reduction glottoplasty (LRG), 158, 177–179
  advantages of, 179
  healing phase, 183
  outcomes, 184, 185
  patient selection, 180
  postoperative management, 183
  preoperative therapy, 180, 181
  primary, 179
  secondary, 179
  staged, 179

surgical techniques, 181, 183
voice assessment
high-speed laryngoscopy and digital kymography, 180
stroboscopy, 179
subjective voice evaluation, 180
voice analysis, 179
Lessac–Madsen Resonant Voice Therapy (LMRVT), 79
“Living full time” requirement, 21

M

Male pitch, 139
Male to female (MTF), 9, 10
Masculinization of voice and communication
generalization of, 147, 148
intonation, pitch variation, and volume, 140
language and nonverbal communication, 141, 142
pitch, 138, 139
resonance and articulation, 139, 140
techniques and strategies for, 142
intonation, pitch variation, and language, 146, 147
pitch, 142–144
resonance, 145, 146
respiration, 147
testosterone on voice, 136, 137
treatment considerations, 149, 150
vocal dissatisfaction in individuals post-testosterone, 137
Microaggression, 28
Microflap elevator, 192
Minority stress model, 33
Misgendering, 38
Modified Isshiki type III, 210
Modified voice, 122, 123
Modified Wendler glottoplasty, 158, 187, 188, 191–194
advantages, 189
drawbacks, 189
outcomes
durability of procedure, 196
healing phase, 195
return to voice procedure, 195
postoperative management, 194, 195
preoperative assessment, 189, 190
preoperative therapy, 190, 191
surgical techniques, 191–193
Motor learning, 84, 149
Muscle tension dysphonia (MTD), 92, 180

N

Nonbinary person, 29
Nonverbal communication, 141, 142
definition of, 103
and gender expression, 105
eye gaze, 106
facial, 105
haptics, 106
kinetics, 106
proxemics, 106
pitfals and considerations
being perspectives, 110
client commitment, 110
clinician personal biases, 109
evolving terminology, 110
rationale for, 104, 105
role of training, 104, 105
situations, 109
techniques, 107–109
Normophonic voicing, 47, 48

O

Oocyte cryopreservation, 8
Orchiectomy, 11

P

Patient-reported outcome measures (PROMs), 44, 45, 48, 49, 163
Phonotrauma, 117
Pitch, 138, 139, 142–144
Pitch-based therapies, 158
Pitch contrast exercise, 93, 94
Pitch in TGNC voice care, 89
Antoni method, 93, 94
recommendations for facilitating to desired pitch, 98, 99
research on, 90, 91
techniques for pitch-based instruction, 95, 96
emotional tone of voice range, 96
lightening the vocal tone, 96
twang voice quality, 97
voice onset practice, 97
Pitch range therapies
research on, 90, 91
in voice modifications, 91, 92
Pitch variation, 140, 146, 147
Pressed phonation, 117
Pre-surgical psychiatric assessment, 18–23
Primary LRG, 179
Puberty-delaying approach, 8
Puberty suppression, 8

Q

Quality of life, 222

R

Registration, 117
Resonance, 145, 146
  and articulation, 139, 140
  definition of, 79
  forward, 81–84
  and pitch contrast exercise, 93, 94
  transgender and gender nonconforming individuals, 81
Resonant voice therapy (RVT), 66, 79, 80
  forward resonance, 81, 83, 84
  pitfalls, 85, 86
  practice and maintenance considerations, 84, 85
  resonance with TGNC individuals, 81
  resonant hum, 82
  transitioning to speaking voice, 83
Respiration, 147
Role-play, 108

S

Secondary LRG, 179
Self-administer reposturing technique, 144
Semi-occluded vocal tract (SOVT), 67, 69, 117, 120
Singing voice, 114, 115
  anxiety and mental health management, 127, 128
  balancing sustainable singing with gender-affirming modification, 125
    laryngeal position, 125
    onset, 125
    tension and functional disruption, 126
    vocal fatigue, 125
    warming up and cooling down, 125
  consultation/vocal counseling, 119
  estrogen-based HRT, 126, 127
  expectation and outcomes, 119, 120
    sample exercises, 123, 124
    social vocal transition, 120
    technical vocal transition, 120–123
  laryngologist, SLP recommendations, and access to care, 129
  rapport-building, 118, 119
Social participation, 49
Social vocal transition, 120
Sound pressure level (SPL), 169
Speaking fundamental frequency (SFF), 90, 91
Speech-language pathologies (SLPs), 31, 43, 103, 104, 107, 108
Sperm banking, 8
Spironolactone, 10, 11
Staged LRG, 179
Straw phonation, 67
Stretch and flow phonation (FP), 66, 69–74
Stretch and flow voice therapy (SnF), 66
Stroboscopy, 179
Subglottal pressure, 117
Subjective voice evaluation, 180
Subplatysmal dissection, 165

T

TA-dominant, 118
Technical vocal transition, 120, 121
  hybrid voice, 122
  modified voice, 122, 123
  unmodified voice, 122
Tessitura, 118
Testosterone, 10, 14, 15, 136, 137, 157
Thin-edge phonation, 118
Thyroarytenoid, 118
Thyroid cartilage reduction, 217
  outcomes, 222
  postoperative management, 221
  preoperative assessment, 217–219
  preoperative therapy, 219
  surgical techniques, 219–221
Thyroid chondroplasty, *see* Thyroid cartilage reduction
Thyroplasties, 177
Trach shave, *see* Thyroid cartilage reduction
Transfeminine voice care, 29
Transgender and gender non-conforming (TGNC)
  individuals, 44, 135
    acoustic, aerodynamic, and auditory-perceptual evaluation, 50, 51
    acoustic/aerodynamic/perceptual analysis for pre- and post-operative gender-affirming voice surgery, 52, 53
    airflow considerations with, 68, 69
    clinician-perceived dysphonia, 46–47
    data collection, 45
    gender-affirming voice targets from cisgender voice norms, limitations of, 51, 52
    Normophonic Voicing, 47, 48
    patient-reported outcomes, 45
    PROMs, 48, 49
    resonance with, 81

voice modification, 27, 39, 40
common issues when interacting with, 38
communities in United States, 30
consent, 35–38
discrimination in healthcare, 31, 32
disparities in health outcomes, 31, 32
language, 28
misgendering, 38
negative feedback, 39
service providers, 30, 31
TIC considerations to institutional settings, 34–36
trauma-informed practice with, 32, 33
voice feminization, 29, 30
Transgender men
hormone regimes, 12
hormone therapy for, 13, 14
Transgender patients, 7
diagnosis and decision to begin treatment, 7, 8
medical management of
adolescents, 8
children, 8
fertility preservation, 8, 9
general health surveillance and screening, 14, 15
hormone therapy, 9–14
perioperative hormone management, 13
Transgender person, 28
Transgender Self-Evaluation Questionnaire (TSEQ), 48, 208
Transgender women, 177
gender affirmimg procedure in, 18
hormone regimes for, 10
hormone therapy for, 9–12
Transsexual Voice Questionnaire (TVQ^{MtF}), 48, 209
Trans Woman Voice Questionnaire (TWVQ), 48, 170
Twang voice quality, 97
Type III thyroplasty, 207, 208, 211–213
informed consent, 209
outcomes, 214
postoperative management, 213, 214
preoperative assessment, 208
preoperative voice therapy, 209
surgical techniques, 210, 211
voice questionnaires, 208, 209

U
Unmodified voice, 122

V
Vaginoplasty, 11
Valuable adjunct role, 31
Visual perception, 107
Vocal dissatisfaction in individuals post-testosterone, 137
Vocal fatigue, 125
Vocal pedagogy, 114
Vocal pitch, 158
Vocal therapy, 18
Voice, characteristics of, 158
Voice feminisation surgery, 164
Voice feminization, 29, 30
Voice Handicap Index (VHI), 48, 49, 170
Voice Handicap Index-10 (VHI-10), 49
Voice masculinization, *see* Masculinization of voice and communication
Voice onset practice, 97
Voice rehabilitation, 65
Voice surgery, 158
Voice therapy, 135

W
Wendler glottoplasty, 52, 187, 188
World Health Organization International Classification of Functioning, Disability, and Health (WHO ICF) model, 43
World Professional Association for Transgender Health (WPATH), 8, 19, 30, 44

GPSR Compliance

The European Union's (EU) General Product Safety Regulation (GPSR) is a set of rules that requires consumer products to be safe and our obligations to ensure this.

If you have any concerns about our products, you can contact us on ProductSafety@springernature.com

In case Publisher is established outside the EU, the EU authorized representative is:

Springer Nature Customer Service Center GmbH
Europaplatz 3
69115 Heidelberg, Germany

Batch number: 10370708

Printed by Printforce, the Netherlands